Test Bank

Audrey J. Berman, PhD, RN, AOCN
Rebecca B. Griffin, RN, MS
Allen M. Hamilton, RN, BSN, MS
Dawna Martich, RN, BSN, MS
Kathryn A. McClure, RN, BSN, MS
Heidi A. Walker, RN, BSN

Fundamentals of Nursing

Concepts, Process, and Practice

Sixth Edition

Barbara Kozier, RN, MN

Glenora Erb, RN, BSN

Audrey Jean Berman, PhD, RN, AOCN
Associate Dean, Nursing Academic Affairs
Samuel Merritt College
Oakland, California

Karen Burke, RN, MS
Director of Health
Clapsop Community College
Astoria, Oregon

Prentice Hall
Upper Saddle River, New Jersey 07458

Publisher: *Julie Alexander*
Editor in Chief: *Cheryl Mehalik*
Acquisitions Editor: *Nancy Anselment*
Cover Design: *Yvo Riezebos Design*
Director of Manufacturing and Production:
   Bruce Johnson
Manufacturing Buyer: *Ilene Sanford*
Managing Editor for Production: *Patrick Walsh*
Printer/Binder: *TK*
Cover Ilustration: The quilt, *Summer's End*, was cre-
ated by Joy Saville and Photographed by William
Taylor.

Previously published by Addison Wesley Nursing
A Division of the Benjamin/Cummings Publishing Company, Inc.
Menlo Park, California 94025

Printed in the United States of America.

ISBN 0-8053-8343-3

10 9 8 7 6 5 4 3 2 1

Prentice-Hall International (UK) Limited, London
Prentice-Hall of Australia Pty. Limited, Sydney
Prentice-Hall Canada Inc., Toronto
Prentice-Hall Hispanoamericana, S. A., Mexico
Prentice-Hall of India Private Limited, New Delhi
Prentice-Hall of Japan, Inc., Tokyo

Care has been taken to confirm the accuracy of information presented in this book. The authors, editors,
and the publisher, however, cannot accept any responsibility for errors or omissions or for the consequences from application of the information in this
book and make no warranty, expressed or implied,
with respect to its contents.

The authors and publisher have exerted every effort to ensure that drug selections and dosages set
forth in this text are in accord with current recommendation and practice at time of publication. However, in view of ongoing research, changes in
government regulations, and the constant flow of information relating to drug therapy and drug reactions, the reader is urged to check the package inserts
of all drugs for any change in indications of dosage
and for added warnings and precautions. This is par-
ticularly important when the recommended agent is a
new and/or infrequently employed drug.

PREFACE

This *Test Bank* to accompany the Sixth Edition of *Fundamentals of Nursing* has been revised and updated with over 250 new multiple-choice questions emphasizing comprehension and application of concepts. It should assist you in testing students with real-life situations that reinforce critical thinking.

The Test Bank offers complete review of the textbook material and provides you with an easy-to-use resource for creating many unique examinations quickly and efficiently. Test items are modeled on the computerized adaptive testing NCLEX format. Each question is completely free-standing; questions do not refer to previously cited scenarios. Where real-life scenarios are used, they are presented entirely within a single question. For each question, students choose one best answer from the four options. The options do not include "all of the above" or "none of the above."

Test items have been coded with the appropriate category: cognitive level, nursing process step, and client needs. Questions are coded with the appropriate type within each category. These categories are divided in the following ways:

Cognitive Level
Knowledge
Comprehension
Application

Nursing Process Steps
Assessment
Analysis/Diagnosis
Planning
Implementation
Evaluation

Client Needs
Safety = Safe, Effective Care Environment
Management of Care
Safety and Infection Control

Promotion = Health Promotion and Maintenance
Growth and Development Through the Life Span
Prevention and Early Detection of Disease

Psychosocial = Psychosocial Integrity
Coping and Adaptation
Psychosocial Adaptation

Physiological = Physiological Integrity
Basic Care and Comfort
Pharmacological and Parenteral Therapies
Reduction of Risk Potential
Physiological Adaptation

Testing aids are offered free to adopters of the textbook in a variety of forms: this printed test bank and its computerized versions; the CD-ROM that accompanies the text; and interactive multiple-choice and essay questions that can be found at the Companion Website for *Fundamentals of Nursing* at http://www.prenhall.com/pubguide.

If you have any questions about testing software, please contact Prentice Hall at at 1-800-677-6337 (8:00 a.m. to 5:00 p.m. M-F CST), or e-mail media.support@pearsoned.com for technical support. The authors, editors, and publishers have sought to provide you with a comprehensive testing package that offers quality test items, flexibility, variety, and accuracy.

Acknowledgments
The authors would like to thank the following reviewers:
Barbara P. Daniel, RN, CS, MEd, MS, Cecil Community College
Candace R. Gioia, RN, BSN, CNOR, Pinellas Technical Education Center(Clearwater Campus
Allen M. Hamilton, RN, BSN, MS, McLennan Community College
Cynthia M. Parsons, RN, MSN, Caldwell Community College
Priscilla L. Sagar, RN, MSN, Dorothea Hopfer School of Nursing at Mount Vernon Hospital

CONTENTS

1   Holistic and Contemporary Nursing Practice

b
Comprehension
Implementation
Safety: Management
of Care

1-1   A common theme contained in definitions of nursing is that nursing is caring that:

a.   involves knowledge about advances in technology.

b.   is concerned with health promotion, maintenance, restoration, and support of the dying.

c.   focuses on the commonalties among individuals and groups.

d.   can benefit either the community or the individual.

c
Knowledge
Safety: Management
of Care

1-2   Nursing organizations must perform which of the following functions for the preservation and development of the profession?

a.   enforce legislative rules and regulations

b.   apply knowledge from the basic sciences

c.   socialize new members to the profession

d.   make provisions for social reforms

b
Comprehension
Safety: Management
of Care

1.3.   Which of the following activities demonstrates nursing autonomy?

a.   receiving direct reimbursement for nursing services

b.   having authority to define nursing functions and roles

c.   establishing a governing board to enforce regulations and laws

d.   creating a professional representative organization

a
Comprehension
Safety: Management
of Care

1-4   Which of the following is characteristic of nursing in ancient civilizations (that is, before 100 B.C.)?

a.   It frequently involved myths, magic and/or religion.

b.   In all societies, it was performed exclusively by women.

c.   Well preserved artifacts provide detailed information about it.

d.   It took place, for the most part, in institutions built by religious orders, such as the Sisters of Charity.

d
Comprehension
Safety: Management
of Care

1-5   What was the significance of the creation of the Institute of Protestant Deaconesses at Kaiserswerth, Germany, in the 1800s?

a.   It marked the beginning of the religious influence on nursing.

b.   It marked the time when women began caring for the sick.

c.   It provided opportunity for prisoners and prostitutes to be rehabilitated as nurses.

d.   It made nursing outside of a religious order an acceptable role for 'proper' women.

d
Comprehension
Safety: Management
of Care

1-6   During which period did rapid reform of nursing services and
       development of planned educational programs occur in North America?

       a.   before the American Revolution (1775 to 1783)

       b.   before the American Civil War

       c.   during the Middle Ages (500 to 1500)

       d.   during the late 1800s

c
Comprehension
Safety: Management
of Care

1-7   According to Miller, which of the following nurses demonstrates
       professional behavior?

       a.   a nurse who graduates from an accredited university school of
            nursing

       b.   a nurse who consistently performs technical skills with flawless
            technique

       c.   a nurse who is active in her/his professional organization (e.g., ANA)

       d.   a nurse who is the supervisor of several nursing units

a
Knowledge
Safety: Management
of Care

1-8   Which of the following is associated with standards of training and
       practice that are determined by the individuals who perform the work?

       a.   profession

       b.   vocation

       c.   occupation

       d.   organization

d
Knowledge
Safety: Management
of Care

1-9   Which of the following recommendations made by the Rockefeller
       Survey played an important role in the historical development of
       nursing?

       a.   Provide planned educational programs for nurses.

       b.   Establish nursing and health services in America.

       c.   Provide more clinical content in nursing programs.

       d.   Move nursing schools out of hospitals and into colleges.

b
Knowledge
Implementation
Psychosocial:
Coping and
Adaptation

1-10   The nurse who assists the client to identify and cope with stressful
       psychological or social problems is functioning in the role of:

       a.   teacher.

       b.   counselor.

       c.   change agent.

       d.   leader.

a
Application
Assessment
Psychosocial:
Coping and
Adaptation

1-11   Realizing that his disease cannot be cured, a client has chosen not to have radiation therapy or further surgery. He has thought carefully about his options. His nurse knows that she would want to fight to the end if she were in his position, but she is able to see the situation through his eyes and understand his feelings. Such sensitivity and awareness are elements of a type of nursing knowledge that Carper calls:

a.   nursing esthetics.

b.   nursing ethics.

c.   nursing science.

d.   personal knowledge.

c
Knowledge
Implementation
Safety: Management
of Care

1-12   A nurse who functions in the role of the client advocate:

a.   makes decisions for the client.

b.   counsels the client about the appropriate decisions.

c.   supports the client's decisions.

d.   shares his or her own preferences with the client.

c
Knowledge
Safety: Management
of Care

1-13   Which of the following is the professional organization that establishes ethical codes and standards of nursing practice in the United States?

a.   National Nurses' Association

b.   National League for Nursing

c.   American Nurses Association

d.   International Council of Nurses

a
Comprehension
Safety: Management
of Care

1-14   According to Benner, the characteristic that separates a 'proficient' nurse from those at lower levels of nursing expertise is:

a.   the ability to understand situations holistically.

b.   an advanced educational preparation.

c.   an intuitive understanding of situations.

d.   the ability to organize.

d
Knowledge
Safety: Management
of Care

1-15   Which of the following nursing roles requires delegated authority within a formal organization?

a.   leader

b.   teacher

c.   communicator/helper

d.   manager

c
Knowledge
Implementation
Safety: Management
of Care

1-16   A nurse who uses interpersonal influence to guide a client in making decisions about her/his health is acting in the role of:

a.   care giver.

b.   communicator.

c.   leader.

d.   advocate.

c
Comprehension
Safety: Management
of Care

1-17   Which of the following is considered to be an expanded nursing role?

a.   staff nurse

b.   nurse aide

c.   clinical nurse specialist

d.   home health nurse

c
Knowledge
Safety: Management
of Care

1-18   The national organization whose objective is to foster the development and improvement of all nursing services and nursing education services in the United States is the:

a.   American Nurses Association.

b.   Sigma Theta Tau.

c.   National League for Nursing.

d.   International Council of Nurses.

a
Knowledge
Safety: Management
of Care

1-19   The first African-American nurse in America was trained:

a.   after the Civil War (in 1879).

b.   during the American Revolution.

c.   after World War I (in 1921).

d.   during World War II (in the 1940s).

c
Comprehension
Safety: Management
of Care

1-20   Standards of clinical nursing practice are:

a.   used as the legal limits of practice.

b.   the policies and procedures that guide nursing practice.

c.   definitions of client outcomes for which nurses are accountable.

d.   suggested guidelines for acute care nursing practice

b
Application
Promotion:
Prevention and Early
Detection of Disease

1-21   As a result of Lillian Wald's work, public health nursing services were initiated in New York City. Today, communities have:

a. professional and social education activities.

b. professional nurses acting in a diversity of settings.

c. health care for the poor.

d. birth control information available in the community.

c
Knowledge
Promotion: Growth
and Development
Through the Life
Span

2-1 The lifelong process by which people learn to become members of society is called:

   a. acculturation.

   b. assimilation.

   c. socialization.

   d. re-socialization.

d
Knowledge
Implementation
Promotion:
Prevention and Early
Detection of Disease

2-2 Which of the following best describes the function of health promotion in nursing practice?

   a. helping people to maintain their present health status

   b. assisting people to improve health following an illness

   c. comforting and caring for people who are dying

   d. helping people to develop resources for maintaining or improving their well-being

a
Knowledge
Safety: Management
of Care

2-3 Individuals prepare to practice as registered nurses by obtaining education in a(n):

   a. baccalaureate nursing program.

   b. inservice education program.

   c. vocational nursing program.

   d. continuing education program.

c
Knowledge
Promotion:
Prevention and Early
Detection of Disease

2-4 A person who collaborates in health care and is responsible for his or her health is defined as a(n):

   a. patient.

   b. consumer.

   c. client.

   d. advocate.

a
Knowledge
Safety: Management
of Care

2-5 Nurse practice acts all have the common purpose of:

   a. protecting the public.

   b. guaranteeing employment.

   c. expanding nursing roles.

   d. assuring national mobility.

a
Knowledge
Safety: Management
of Care

2-6 Which of the following is a function of the standards of nursing practice formulated by professional nursing organizations?

a. define professional accountability to the public

b. establish legislative regulations

c. differentiate advanced practitioners from novices

d. provide for career mobility

b
Knowledge
Safety: Management
of Care

2-7 Which of the following is intended to guarantee minimum standards for credentialing, or entry into the nursing profession?

a. standards of clinical nursing practice

b. state nurse practice acts

c. the Patient Self-Determination Act

d. federal laws

c
Application
Safety: Management
of Care

2-8 Horizontal career mobility is best described as:

a. changing from a staff nurse to unit supervisor position.

b. changing from a staff nurse to nurse practitioner position.

c. moving from a medical ward to a mental health unit.

d. getting a masters degree in nursing.

c
Comprehension
Safety: Management
of Care

2-9 The increasing proportion of very ill clients in hospitals and the shift from hospital to home-based care has been primarily caused by:

a. use of diagnostic related groups (DRGs) in medical records.

b. the nursing shortage of the 1990s.

c. limits on lengths of stay by health maintenance organizations (HMOs).

d. the large number of people with acquired immune deficiency syndrome (AIDS).

a
Comprehension
Implementation
Safety: Management
of Care

2-10 Nurses entering practice today should expect to:

a. give specialized care using sophisticated techniques and technology.

b. encounter consumers who are less vocal about their health care needs.

c. care for a decreasing proportion of elderly clients in the next five years.

d. follow the population shift to rural settings.

a
Knowledge
Safety: Management
of Care

2-11 Which of the following factors has been influential in raising the autonomy and group consciousness of nurses?

    a.   the women's movement

    b.   the nursing shortage of the 1980s

    c.   the National Commission on Nursing Implementation Project (NCNIP)

    d.   recent changes in licensure laws

b
Knowledge
Safety: Management
of Care

2-12 Continuing education programs are designed to help practicing nurses:

    a.   review basic information essential to their clinical practice.

    b.   update skills and information related to their area of expertise.

    c.   renew their nursing license.

    d.   socialize within the profession.

b
Comprehension
Safety: Management
of Care

2-13 To respond to new knowledge and societal trends, how have nursing curricula changed in the past few years?

    a.   more emphasis on pathophysiology, pharmacology, and treatment of diseases

    b.   greater focus on critical thinking and application of knowledge rather than memorization of facts

    c.   a return to learning by observation and experience (apprenticeship training)

    d.   increased amount of time spent on the skills needed to practice in the hospital setting

c
Knowledge
Safety: Management
of Care

2-14 What level of education do the American Nurses Association and the Canadian Nurses Association recommend as the entry level for professional nursing practice?

    a.   education in a vocational nursing program

    b.   education in an associate degree nursing program

    c.   a baccalaureate degree in nursing

    d.   a baccalaureate degree in any science

b
Knowledge
Safety: Management
of Care

2-15 Under state laws in the United States and Canada, who is recognized as a nurse?

    a.   only registered nurses (RNs)

    b.   both registered nurses (RNs) and practical/vocational nurses (LPNs or LVNs)

    c.   only RNs with a baccalaureate degree

    d.   nurses with associate and/or baccalaureate degrees, but not diploma degrees

c
Knowledge
Safety: Management
of Care

2-16   What is the primary problem with the associate degree education of nurses pioneered by Mildred Montag?

   a.   The schools are not subject to accreditation by the National League for Nurses.

   b.   Students do not take college level courses, so they cannot write the RN national licensing exam.

   c.   Graduates are not used by hospitals in the manner intended by Montag.

   d.   The program of study is too long and difficult for most students.

c
Comprehension
Safety: Management
of Care

2-17   A nurse is attending a review of cardiopulmonary resuscitation (CPR) offered and required by the nursing home where she works. What type of education is this is an example of?

   a.   professional

   b.   continuing

   c.   inservice

   d.   advanced

a
Application
Safety: Management
of Care

2-18   An instructor asks her students to take part in a research project by allowing her to measure their height and weight. The instructor says it isn't a course requirement, but that she would really appreciate their participation. Which human subjects right is at greatest risk of being violated in this situation?

   a.   right to self-determination

   b.   right to disclosure

   c.   right to privacy

   d.   right to not be harmed

d
Comprehension
Safety: Management
of Care

2-19   If you needed money for nursing research, you would want to know which research priorities were currently being funded. Where would you go to obtain this information?

   a.   National League for Nursing

   b.   American or Canadian Nurses Association

   c.   Sigma Theta Tau

   d.   Institute for Nursing Research

a
Knowledge
Safety: Management
of Care

2-20   Credentialing for expanded practice roles such as nurse anesthesia is carried out by the:

   a.   American Nurses Association or nursing specialty organizations.

   b.   state boards of nursing.

   c.   National League for Nursing.

   d.   National Commission on Nursing Implementation Project.

b
Application
Safety: Management
of Care

2-21   Vertical career mobility may be described as:

    a.   changing from a medical unit to a surgical unit.

    b.   changing from a staff nurse to nurse manager position.

    c.   moving from a nurse manager to clinical nurse specialist position.

    d.   moving from a nurse educator to nurse researcher position.

c
Comprehension
Safety: Management
of Care

2-22   Polit and Hungler provide several rationales for the importance of nursing research. Which of the following rationales would have the most impact on nursing at the bedside?

    a.   Nursing research expands the scientific body of knowledge.

    b.   Research by nurses increases the accountability to general public.

    c.   Research can demonstrate the efficacy of nursing interventions.

    d.   Nursing research identifies the best intervention for each clinical situation.

d
Knowledge
Safety: Management
of Care

2-23   A nurse who critically analyzes or critiques nursing research should examine many areas. Which of the following aspects of research has the greatest significance?

    a.   theoretical framework

    b.   nursing model and methodology

    c.   the ethical dimensions

    d.   the interpretation of results and application to practice

a
Knowledge
Safety: Management
of Care

2-24   According to the *Guidelines for the Investigative Functions of Nurses* (ANA), the associate degree nurse is able to:

    a.   collect data within an established research project.

    b.   apply the findings of nursing research to nursing practice.

    c.   conduct investigations that monitor the quality of clinical practice.

    d.   develop methods to investigate physiological phenomena.

3   NURSING THEORIES AND CONCEPTUAL FRAMEWORKS

d
Knowledge
Safety: Management
of Care

3-1   How is a theory different from a conceptual framework?

    a.   A theory may contain constructs.

    b.   A theory is made up of concepts and propositions.

    c.   A theory includes testable propositions.

    d.   A theory is more abstract and less specific than a conceptual model.

c
Knowledge
Safety: Management
of Care

3-2   The best definition of a conceptual model is a(n):

    a.   pattern or abstract outline of something.

    b.   abstract idea that provides a representation of reality.

    c.   set of statements that expresses the relationships between ideas about reality.

    d.   set of statements that generates knowledge in a field.

a
Knowledge
Safety: Management
of Care

3-3   The individual who believed to be the first nurse theorist is:

    a.   Florence Nightingale.

    b.   Virginia Henderson.

    c.   Martha Rogers.

    d.   Sr. Callista Roy.

b
Knowledge
Promotion:
Prevention and Early
Detection of Disease

3-4   Nursing theories should include descriptions of the four metaparadigm concepts. Those concepts are:

    a.   person, society, wellness, and illness.

    b.   person, environment, health/illness, and nursing.

    c.   nursing, environment, health, and illness.

    d.   nursing, environment, person, and society.

c
Application
Psychosocial:
Psychosocial
Adaptation

3-5   A nursing theory or model that focuses on communication and relationships between people is considered to be of the _____ type.

    a.   developmental

    b.   systems

    c.   interactional

    d.   environmental

a
Knowledge
Safety: Management
of Care

3-6   A _____ is an abstract image or idea of reality, usually represented by a word, which brings forth mental pictures of the properties and meanings of things.

a. concept
b. theory
c. proposition
d. model

a
Comprehension
Promotion:
Prevention and Early
Detection of Disease

3-7   In Orem's nursing model, the role of the nurse is to:

a. influence the client's development in achieving an optimal level of self-care.
b. promote the client's adaptive behaviors by manipulating stimuli.
c. identify and help the individual respond to stressors.
d. help clients develop patterns of living that accommodate environmental changes.

c
Knowledge
Planning
Promotion:
Prevention and Early
Detection of Disease

3-8   Maintenance of system equilibrium is a goal of:

a. Dorothy Johnson's behavioral systems model.
b. Rosemarie Parse's human-living-health model.
c. Betty Neuman's health care systems model.
d. Imogene King's systems interaction model.

a
Comprehension
Safety: Management
of Care

3-9   Which of the following is a good reason for advocating a single, universal model for nursing?

a. It would provide a common framework for all nurses, thereby enhancing communication.
b. It would allow nurses to examine phenomena in different ways and from different viewpoints.
c. It would foster development of the full scope and potential of nursing.
d. It would bring nursing to the level of other professions.

b
Comprehension
Safety: Management
of Care

3-10   What is the relationship between the nursing process and nursing models?

a. The nursing process is one of the major units making up all nursing models.
b. The nursing process is the method by which nursing models are put into practice.
c. The nursing process is a problem-solving process that is unrelated to nursing models.
d. The nursing process is a systematic process used to develop nursing models.

a
Comprehension
Promotion:
Prevention and Early
Detection of Disease

3-11   The theories of Roy, King, Neuman, and Johnson are all systems theories. A common thread running through any systems theory is the idea of:

a.   interrelated parts functioning together to form the whole.

b.   a whole that is made up of independently functioning parts.

c.   stability, lack of movement, or change.

d.   clear barriers separating systems from each other.

d
Knowledge
Promotion:
Prevention and Early
Detection of Disease

3-12   'Input' in Roy's Adaptation Model (a systems model) refers to:

a.   a process of transformation.

b.   a process by which a system regulates itself.

c.   sets of interacting, identifiable components.

d.   internal and external stimuli the individual receives.

a
Knowledge
Promotion:
Prevention and Early
Detection of Disease

3-13   According to Leininger's care theory, caring values and behaviors are derived largely from a person's:

a.   culture.

b.   experience.

c.   education.

d.   occupation.

b
Knowledge
Implementation
Promotion:
Prevention and Early
Detection of Disease

3-14   Benner identifies six qualities of power associated with caring. Which of these qualities is demonstrated by a nurse who acts on behalf of clients and families?

a.   integrative caring power

b.   advocacy power

c.   healing power

d.   transformative power

a
Application
Implementation
Promotion:
Prevention and Early
Detection of Disease

3-15   Which nursing activity best demonstrates application of the Nightingale theory of nursing?

a.   working with a community group to improve air quality in the city

b.   taking a client to the chapel in a wheelchair

c.   manipulating a client's energy fields through therapeutic touch

d.   focusing on communication and mutual goal setting

c
Comprehension
Safety: Management
of Care

3-16   Theory is useful for nursing practice, education, and research. A nurse researcher would be most likely to use theory to:

a.   narrow the supporting literature to that most relevant.

b.   guide criteria to evaluate the quality of nursing care in an institution.

c.   identify knowledge gaps in nursing.

d.   justify research as an appropriate nursing role.

a
Knowledge
Promotion:
Prevention and Early
Detection of Disease

3-17　The 'goal of nursing' is an important element in all nursing models. Which theorist believes that the goal of nursing is to make the client comfortable and put the client in the best possible condition to allow nature to act?

a.　Florence Nightingale

b.　Virginia Henderson

c.　Jean Watson

d.　Imogene King

d
Application
Psychosocial:
Coping and
Adaptation

3-18　"When stressors make it impossible for the person to cope, then the person needs a nurse." This is an example of a(n):

a.　concept.

b.　construct.

c.　hypothesis.

d.　proposition.

c
Application
Promotion:
Prevention and Early
Detection of Disease

3-19　Evaluate the following nursing theory: "Nursing interventions are performed within the context of the nursing process. They involve manipulating stimuli to support and promote independent functioning of the client, a biopsychosocial being." Which of the four major concepts is missing or least developed?

a.　person/client

b.　environment

c.　health/illness

d.　nursing

a
Comprehension
Psychosocial:
Psychosocial
Adaptation

3-20　In caring theories, the central emphasis is on:

a.　the nurse-client relationship and psychosocial aspects of care.

b.　pathophysiology and self-care abilities.

c.　maintaining client balance or homeostasis.

d.　compensating for client deficits.

c
Knowledge
Promotion:
Prevention and Early
Detection of Disease

3-21　In holistic theory, which of the following describes the relationship of the parts of a living organism to the whole organism?

a.　The sum of the parts is equal to the whole.

b.　The sum of the parts is greater than the whole.

c.　The whole is greater than the sum of the parts.

d.　The sum of the parts is not related to the whole.

b
Application
Safety: Management
of Care

4-1   Which of the following statements accurately reflects the nurse's legal liability for delegating to unlicensed assistive personnel (UAP)?

    a.   The nurse is liable for any and all actions performed by the UAP.

    b.   The nurse may legally delegate tasks but not the nursing process to the UAP.

    c.   The nurse is not liable for any of the UAPs actions.

    d.   The nurse is liable only for those actions that the nurse directly observes the UAP performing.

a
Knowledge
Implementation
Safety: Management
of Care

4-2   One function of the law in nursing is to:

    a.   help determine the boundaries of independent nursing action.

    b.   assure comparable reimbursement for services.

    c.   define the standards of professional practice.

    d.   differentiate between ethical and unethical practice.

b
Comprehension
Safety: Management
of Care

4-3   The purpose of the Patient Self-Determination Act is to permit clients to:

    a.   ensure that health care workers do what the client wants.

    b.   delineate health care choices in case they are later unable to do so themselves.

    c.   identify how, when, and where they wish to die.

    d.   prevent health care workers from trying experimental procedures without the client's express consent.

b
Knowledge
Safety: Management
of Care

4-4   The body of law that deals with relationships between private individuals is termed:

    a.   public law.

    b.   civil law.

    c.   common law.

    d.   criminal law.

d
Comprehension
Safety: Management
of Care

4-5   Which of the following categories of law deals with libel and slander?

    a.   statutory

    b.   criminal

    c.   contracts

    d.   torts

a
Knowledge
Safety: Management
of Care

4-6 Which of the following is a responsibility of state boards of nursing in the United States?

a. examining and licensing of qualified candidates

b. setting standards for professional practice

c. conducting trials of nurses accused of criminal acts

d. collective bargaining

c
Comprehension
Safety: Management
of Care

4-7 In order to prove that nursing malpractice has occurred, the plaintiff must prove that the nurse:

a. intended to harm the client.

b. carries malpractice insurance.

c. acted outside care standards.

d. had performed that action safely previously.

a
Knowledge
Safety: Management
of Care

4-8 Nursing licensure for registered nurses in the United States is:

a. mandatory.

b. permissive.

c. federal.

d. institutional.

b
Knowledge
Safety: Management
of Care

4-9 Nursing licensure for registered nurses in Canada is:

a. mandatory in all provinces.

b. mandatory in most provinces.

c. not mandatory in any provinces.

d. mandatory in only a few provinces.

c
Knowledge
Safety: Management
of Care

4-10 Individuals have a right to withhold themselves and their lives from public scrutiny. The intentional tort that results from not respecting this right is termed:

a. slander.

b. false imprisonment.

c. invasion of privacy.

d. battery.

d
Knowledge
Implementation
Safety: Management
of Care

4-11 An attempt or threat to touch another person unjustifiably describes the intentional tort of:

a. libel.

b. slander.

c. false imprisonment.

d. assault.

b
Application
Evaluation
Safety: Management
of Care

4-12 Two student nurses are eating lunch in the cafeteria, and one of them states that her client is a prostitute, which is why the client contracted genital herpes. In fact, the client is not a prostitute. A close friend of the client is eating lunch at the next table and overhears the conversation. The student nurses may be guilty of:

a. libel.
b. slander.
c. battery.
d. assault.

a
Application
Assessment
Safety: Management
of Care

4-13 During an interview, a nurse writes in her notes that she suspects the client is taking illegal drugs. She misplaces her notepad and the client's family finds it. The nurse could be sued for:

a. libel.
b. slander.
c. negligence.
d. malpractice.

d
Application
Implementation
Safety: Management
of Care

4-14 A nurse is giving medications to a group of clients. He mixes up the medications of two of the clients and gives the wrong drugs. One of the clients has to have her stomach pumped after the incident and almost dies. The nurse could be guilty of:

a. attempted murder.
b. fraud.
c. assault.
d. malpractice.

a
Comprehension
Implementation
Safety: Management
of Care

4-15 Informed consent is defined as:

a. an agreement by the client to accept a course of treatment or procedure after receiving complete information.
b. a legal form that is signed by the client that becomes a permanent part of the chart.
c. a process whereby the client is given an option of several different treatment modalities.
d. a form that contains a description of the procedure or treatment and risks that the nurse explains to the client.

c
Application
Implementation
Safety: Management
of Care

4-16 Which of the following clients *cannot* legally give informed consent?

a. a married, 14-year-old girl

b. a 70-year-old man who is alert and oriented but unable to write his name

c. a 40-year-old client who has been sedated

d. a 50-year-old woman who cannot stop crying during the explanation

b
Knowledge
Evaluation
Safety: Management
of Care

4-17 A primary purpose of an incident report is to:

a. provide evidence for a trial.

b. identify ways to prevent future incidents.

c. identify the person(s) responsible for the incident.

d. assure that necessary follow-up procedures were followed.

a
Knowledge
Implementation
Safety: Management
of Care

4-18 The most common situation for which nurses are charged with malpractice is:

a. making a medication error.

b. not following a physician's order.

c. loss of client property.

d. failure to obtain informed consent.

d
Application
Implementation
Safety: Management
of Care

4-19 The physician has written a DNR (do not resuscitate) order for a client. It is against the nurse's religious beliefs to carry out a DNR order. What should she do?

a. Call the physician and request that he change the order.

b. Talk to the client's family and explain that she will not be able to follow the order.

c. Do nothing, but if the client goes into arrest, go ahead and resuscitate him.

d. Request that the client be assigned to another nurse.

c
Knowledge
Safety: Management
of Care

4-20 Should nurses have their own liability insurance?

a. No, because they are covered under the employer's insurance.

b. No, because they would then be more likely to be sued.

c. Yes, because employer insurance may not cover all the nurse's activities.

d. Yes, because it is not very expensive.

a
Application
Implementation
Safety: Management
of Care

4-21 The medical order reads: 'Nothing by mouth.' However, the client says she is "starving and must have something to eat—or at least to drink." The nurse is aware that most clients having the same surgery are started on clear liquids within 4 hours. The client is already nearly 36 hours post-op, has good bowel sounds, and seems ready for a clear liquid diet. It is 10:30 P.M., what should the nurse do?

a. Call the physician and relay the client's status and request.

b. Give the client a few ice chips or sips of water; if she tolerates that, let her have tea and gelatin.

c. Tell the client that she will "look the other way" if she wants to get a soda from the pantry.

d. Tell the client she will have to wait until morning when the physician makes rounds.

c
Knowledge
Safety: Management
of Care

4-22 The process of formal negotiation of working conditions between groups of RNs and employers is referred to as:

a. a grievance.

b. a strike.

c. collective bargaining.

d. arbitration.

b
Knowledge
Safety: Management
of Care

4-23 Compared to an RN, the student nurse is held to a legal standard:

a. higher than an RN.

b. the same as an RN.

c. less than an RN.

d. leveled depending upon term in the nursing program.

c
Knowledge
Safety: Management
of Care

4-24 Good Samaritan acts protect nurses from liability for acts performed in an emergency situation:

a. no matter what they do.

b. if they have the client's consent.

c. if they are not grossly negligent in their actions.

d. if the client has a good outcome from their actions.

ETHICS, VALUES, AND ADVOCACY

a
Comprehension
Safety: Management
of Care

5-1   With regard to ethical situations in client care, the most important nursing responsibility is to:

    a.   be accountable for the morality of one's own actions.

    b.   remain neutral and fair in ethical decisions.

    c.   realize that the physician is responsible for deciding ethical questions.

    d.   act only when absolutely certain the action is ethically correct.

b
Application
Safety: Management
of Care

5-2   Which of the following is most clearly a question of nursing ethics?

    a.   The nurse is asked to assist in circumcision of newborn male infants. However, there is literature both to support and refute the value of this practice.

    b.   At a party, a nurse overhears her colleagues laughing and talking about one of the clients.

    c.   The nurses on the unit all agree to sign a petition stating they are not paid enough to compensate for the amount of responsibility they have.

    d   A client is unsure about the foods allowed on his low-fat diet and asks the nurse what he should eat.

a
Comprehension
Planning
Safety: Management
of Care

5-3   Nurses can best improve the quality of their ethical decisions by:

    a.   thinking in advance about such dilemmas and how they might handle them.

    b.   taking college or continuing education ethics courses.

    c.   reading and following the ANA *Code of Ethics*.

    d.   knowing and obeying state laws and hospital policies.

b
Comprehension
Implementation
Safety: Management
of Care

5-4   The ANA Code of Ethics indicates that nurses should be client advocates. Advocacy may be difficult for nurses because:

    a.   the Code of Ethics has no religious foundation.

    b.   nurses often do not have the autonomy to act as the client's advocate.

    c.   advocacy conflicts with the utilitarian values of nursing.

    d.   nurses do not have the knowledge to be client advocates.

c
Application
Safety: Management
of Care

5-5   Which of the following represents a potential nursing ethical dilemma?

    a.   "The law says . . ."

    b.   "The client wants . . ."

    c.   "I feel I should . . ."

    d.   "What we usually do is . . ."

5-6 Which type of moral problem involves a difficult decision with no really 'good' answer?

a. moral uncertainty

b. moral dilemma

c. moral distress

d. moral conflict

5-7 Institutional constraints that prevent nurses from carrying out their moral decisions represent which type of moral problem?

a. moral uncertainty

b. moral dilemma

c. moral distress

d. moral outrage

5-8 "People inherently know what is right or wrong; it is not a matter of rational thought or of learning." This statement best defines the moral framework of:

a. teleology.

b. deontology.

c. intuitionism.

d. caring.

5-9 A nurse who is faced with an ethical decision thinks, "If I tell the client the truth, he will be upset; if I don't, he won't have the information he needs to make a good decision about his health." Which framework is the nurse using?

a. teleology

b. deontology

c. intuitionism

d. caring

5-10 A nurse who is making a decision thinks, "I have a duty to do this no matter what happens as a result. This is my moral obligation." Which moral framework is the nurse using?

a. teleology

b. deontology

c. intuitionism

d. caring

d
Application
Safety: Management
of Care

5-11   A nurse who is making an ethical decision primarily thinks about how it
will affect his relationship with his client. He also wishes to maintain the
client's relationships with her family and other caregivers. The nurse is
most likely using the moral framework of:

a. teleology.

b. deontology.

c. intuitionism.

d. caring.

a
Application
Implementation
Safety: Management
of Care

5-12   A client's cancer is very advanced. She has decided not to have surgery or
chemotherapy. Her nurse believes that, as a rule, everything possible
should be done to preserve life. However, once the client has decided, the
nurse supports her decision. Which moral principle provides the best
basis for the nurse's actions?

a. respect for autonomy

b. nonmaleficence

c. beneficence

d. justice

c
Knowledge
Safety: Management
of Care

5-13   The term *beneficence* means:

a. do no harm.

b. fairness.

c. doing good.

d. personal liberty.

a
Application
Safety: Management
of Care

5-14   The nurses on a hospital unit are concerned that one of their colleagues is
not keeping up with information on new medications. One nurse says,
"Nurses ought not be allowed to work if they are not competent." This
statement reflects:

a. a conventional moral principle of nursing.

b. the principle of autonomy.

c. the moral framework of caring.

d. the principle of beneficence.

b
Knowledge
Safety: Management
of Care

5-15   A *code of ethics* is best defined as:

a. a set of values to which one is personally committed.

b. formal guidelines and standards for professional actions.

c. a statement of minimum standards of competent practice.

d. guidelines to which members of the profession are legally bound.

c
Comprehension
Safety: Management
of Care

5-16   Nursing codes of ethics fulfill which of the following purposes?

a.   They define the roles of the nurse, the client, other health care providers, and society.

b.   They define the scope of nursing practice on a national level.

c.   They help the public to understand professional nursing conduct.

d.   They outline actions to be implemented in specific nursing care situations.

b
Application
Assessment
Safety: Management
of Care

5-17   Which of the following statements by the nurse would be most helpful in assisting clients to clarify their values?

a.   "That was not a good decision. Why did you think it would work?"

b.   "Some people might have chosen another way. What led you to make your decision?"

c.   "Your doctor told you what to do. Did you do that?"

d.   "I would have made a different decision. How do you feel about your choice?"

a
Application
Safety: Management
of Care

5-18   Which of the following situations best illustrates values transmission by modeling?

a.   A child imitates his mother's respectful actions toward elderly persons.

b.   A police candidate attends a lecture by the academy trainers regarding values of the police role.

c.   A new member of an organization is provided with a code of 'right' actions.

d.   A political leader delineates values to be taught to all school children.

c
Knowledge
Safety: Management
of Care

5-19   The rules or principles that govern right conduct concerning life, biology, and the health professions are called:

a.   morality.

b.   moral behavior.

c.   bioethics.

d.   values.

d
Comprehension
Safety: Management
of Care

5-20   What do codes of ethics and various ethical decision-making models have in common?

a.   They enable the nurse to function according to legal statutes.

b.   They allow the nurse to function with a clear conscience in ethical situations.

c.   They do not help the nurse to defend her/his moral actions to others.

d.   They do not guarantee that the 'right' decision will be made in a given situation.

b
Application
Intervention
Safety: Management
of Care

5-21 The parents of a genetically impaired newborn have decided not to have the infant treated. The physician, however, is insisting on trying an experimental treatment. The parents look to the nurse for help. Which of the following demonstrates a utilitarian framework perspective?

a. "You ought to do what the doctor says, he knows best."

b. "Maybe the baby's participation will someday benefit other babies."

c. "If you don't agree, the doctor may ask the court to allow it anyway."

d. "There is always hope; it is wrong not to try."

a
Application
Safety: Management
of Care

5-22 An 85-year-old man is refusing dialysis for his kidney failure. The primary ethical principle involved is:

a. autonomy.

b. beneficence.

c. nonmaleficence.

d. justice.

a
Knowledge
Safety: Management
of Care

5-23 According to the deontological approach to bioethics:

a. the ethics of the act is separate from the outcome.

b. the end justifies the means.

c. people automatically know what is good or bad.

d. what the person wants is always the best action.

b
Application
Planning
Safety: Management
of Care

5-24 Your client has recently returned from major surgery with general anesthesia. You intend to turn him but decide not to because it would cause him great pain. You are functioning under the principle of:

a. veracity.

b. nonmaleficence.

c. beneficence.

d. advocacy.

b
Application
Safety: Management
of Care

6.1.   A hospital provides mainly _____ health care.

a.   primary

b.   secondary

c.   tertiary

d.   quaternary

c
Knowledge
Promotion:
Prevention and Early
Detection of Disease

6-2   A purpose of primary health care is to:

a.   provide long-term care.

b.   provide rehabilitative care.

c.   prevent diseases.

d.   provide specialized services.

a
Knowledge
Safety: Management
of Care

6-3   Reimbursement for hospital services is made according to a classification system known as:

a.   diagnosis-related groups.

b.   standards of practice.

c.   state peer review organizations.

d.   health maintenance organizations.

d
Application
Planning
Safety: Management
of Care

6-4   A 65-year-old grandmother who is usually healthy has been experiencing fatigue and difficulty breathing for the past three days. Her family noticed the change in her health and encouraged her to seek medical attention. At this time, the most appropriate care agency for her would be a:

a.   hospice.

b.   hospital.

c.   rehabilitation center.

d.   primary health care provider.

a
Comprehension
Planning
Safety: Management
of Care

6-5   A client is concerned because he does not think he can pay his hospital bill. To assist with this problem, the nurse should notify a:

a.   social worker.

b.   physician.

c.   bookkeeping department.

d.   case manager.

c
Knowledge
Promotion: Growth
and Development
Through the Life
Span

6-6   For most clients over age 65, the majority of their health care costs are provided for by:

    a.   Supplemental Security Income.

    b.   Blue Cross and Blue Shield.

    c.   Medicare.

    d.   Medicaid.

b
Knowledge
Safety: Management
of Care

6-7   In general, what effect does the prospective payment system have on clients' hospitalizations?

    a.   improved medical care

    b.   shorter hospital stays

    c.   longer hospital stays

    d.   more individualized nursing care

c
Comprehension
Implementation
Psychosocial:
Coping and
Adaptation

6-8   A client has been diagnosed as having lung cancer. He has agreed to undergo chemotherapy. How might a self-help group like the American Cancer Society help him?

    a.   Assist with chemotherapy.

    b.   Provide financial assistance.

    c.   Provide emotional support.

    d.   Assist with research activities.

a
Comprehension
Implementation
Safety: Management
of Care

6-9   A client needs a low-fat, low-salt diet because of his hypertension. He should be referred to a:

    a.   dietitian.

    b.   nutritionist.

    c.   physician.

    d.   paramedical technologist.

a
Comprehension
Planning
Psychosocial:
Coping and
Adaptation

6-10   The physical condition of a client who is considered terminally ill is deteriorating rapidly. The nurse wants to refer the client to an organization that provides special care for dying people. Such an organization is:

    a.   a hospice.

    b.   the Veterans Administration.

    c.   a community health center.

    d.   a health maintenance organization.

b
Knowledge
Safety: Management
of Care

6-11 Hospitals have changed greatly in the past 10 years. One such change is that:

a. they now provide mostly outpatient and primary services.

b. the proportion of very ill and elderly clients has increased.

c. large hospitals have stopped offering specialized services.

d. small, rural hospitals have begun to offer an increasingly complex range of services.

a
Knowledge
Safety: Management
of Care

6-12 A health maintenance organization differs from a preferred provider organization in that HMOs:

a. stress wellness, health promotion, and illness prevention.

b. provide services to an insurance company at a discounted rate.

c. charge the client according to the kind of services received.

d. allow clients to choose from among the physicians and hospitals belonging to the organization.

c
Comprehension
Planning
Safety: Management
of Care

6-13 A major purpose of home health care is to:

a. assess health care needs.

b. prevent illness.

c. maximize independent functioning.

d. help clients cope with an immediate crisis.

d
Application
Safety: Management
of Care

6-14 It is anticipated that changes in the health care system will include more emphasis on illness prevention instead of illness treatment. How will this affect the education of future nurses?

a. They will need more in-hospital training.

b. They will need more theory-based education.

c. They will need more research courses.

d. They will need more emphasis on community health.

c
Comprehension
Assessment
Promotion:
Prevention and Early
Detection of Disease

6-15 Which one of the following factors contributes to the poor health of many homeless people?:

a. lack of appreciation for a health lifestyle

b. lack of motivation to seek health care

c. lack of access to health care services

d. lack of awareness of their illness symptoms

c
Application
Implementation
Safety: Management
of Care

6-16　A client who has colon cancer recently underwent a bowel resection with formation of a permanent colostomy. There is an order for colostomy irrigation q.o.d. Two nursing students wish to observe another fellow student performing the irrigation. It is most important for them to ask for the consent of the:

a. charge nurse.

b. physician.

c. client.

d. nursing instructor.

a
Knowledge
Promotion: Growth
and Development
Through the Life
Span

6-17　Which characteristic of families in North America is presently causing stress to the health care delivery system?

a. increase in the number of single parent families

b. increase in the number of families in which both parents work outside the home

c. decrease in the number of children

d. decrease in the number of teenage marriages

b
Comprehension
Promotion: Growth
and Development
Through the Life
Span

6-18　How does the increasing proportion of older adults to younger adults impact the health care system?

a. Older adults have more accidents than other age groups.

b. Older adults have more long-term illnesses than other age groups.

c. Over 30 percent of older adults are institutionalized because of their health problems.

d. Older adults do not benefit much from home care.

a
Knowledge
Safety: Management
of Care

6-19　Critical pathways are most useful for:

a. conditions that are seen frequently in an agency.

b. complex or unusual diseases.

c. clients who require care across a variety of settings.

d. clients with emergency conditions, whose outcomes cannot be predicted.

b
Comprehension
Promotion:
Prevention and Early
Detection of Disease

6-20　A client goes to the local shopping mall for his annual flu shot. What form of health care is this?

a. quaternary

b. tertiary

c. secondary

d. primary

b
Application
Implementation
Psychosocial:
Coping and
Adaptation

6-21   A client's mother is in the early stages of Alzheimer's disease. He is reluctant to institutionalize his parent at this time. The best method of care for his mother would be:

a. daily visits by a public health nurse.

b. adult day care.

c. admission to a long-term care facility.

d. admission to an acute care facility.

d
Comprehension
Safety: Management
of Care

6-22   A client has been diagnosed as terminally ill with metastatic liver cancer. The oncologist recommends aggressive chemotherapy. The client has refused this therapy. His right to refuse treatment is protected by:

a. state health care laws.

b. self-determination laws.

c. informed consent.

d. Patient's Bill of Rights.

d
Knowledge
Safety: Safety and
Infection Control

6-23   Surveillance of infectious diseases is governed by:

a. provincial or state governments.

b. National Institutes of Health.

c. public health services.

d. Centers for Disease Control and Prevention.

b
Application
Safety: Management
of Care

6-24   The RN team leader is legally responsible for:

a. administering all medications.

b. delegating tasks within the legal limitations of practice for the LVN.

c. giving report to the next shift team leader.

d. the competency of the team members.

c
Knowledge
Safety: Management
of Care

6-25   The case manager for the oncology unit is a professional nurse responsible for:

a. arranging home care.

b. assisting with financial arrangements.

c. coordinating all aspects of client care.

d. prescribing client outcomes.

7 COMMUNITY-BASED NURSING AND CARE CONTINUITY

b
Comprehension
Planning
Safety: Management
of Care

7-1 Which of the following identifies a way in which nurses are impacting health care reform?

    a. providing expert assessment skills

    b. adding their presence to a variety of settings

    c. speaking out on health care legislature

    d. providing expert evaluation skills

a
Knowledge
Planning
Safety: Management
of Care

7-2 Which of the following is a characteristic of primary health care?

    a. Community participation is client-directed.

    b. Collaboration occurs among members of the health care team.

    c. Focus is on individuals and families.

    d. Empowerment is a provider-assisted process.

c
Knowledge
Planning
Safety: Management
of Care

7-3 Which of the following is true of nursing's agenda for health care reform?

    a. Essential services will be introduced in the beginning.

    b. Health care cost reduction is not a part of the agenda.

    c. Long-term care provision is essential.

    d. Case management is not a part of the agenda.

b
Knowledge
Planning
Safety: Management
of Care

7-4 Which of the following trends is included in the NLN's 1992 document for health care?

    a. Acute care facilities will expand and become more available to the consumer.

    b. Home care will become the center of health care.

    c. Nurses will find more employment in acute care settings.

    d. Outpatient wellness centers will become the center of health care.

c
Application
Planning
Promotion:
Prevention and Early
Detection of Disease

7-5 Which of the following identifies a similarity between primary health care and primary care?

    a. Both are expert-driven.

    b. Health professionals advise individuals about what is best for their health.

    c. Both strive for universal access and affordability of health care.

    d. Both support a top-down approach to providing health care.

c
Application
Planning
Safety: Management
of Care

7-6   Which of the following is needed for an effective community-based
       health care system?

       a.   well-trained physicians
       b.   well-trained nurses
       c.   easy access
       d.   strong client focus

a
Knowledge
Planning
Promotion:
Prevention and Early
Detection of Disease

7-7   A health care system that provides all levels of care in order to
       facilitate positive health outcomes through health promotion and
       disease prevention is termed:

       a.   an integrated health care system.
       b.   a community initiative.
       c.   managed care.
       d.   case management.

c
Application
Planning
Promotion:
Prevention and Early
Detection of Disease

7-8   The nurse in the community is creating a program to address annual
       flu inoculations and elder abuse. This program is an example of:

       a.   a community initiative.
       b.   managed care.
       c.   a community coalition.
       d.   a lay health worker outreach program.

d
Knowledge
Planning
Promotion:
Prevention and Early
Detection of Disease

7-9   The method to provide health care services to clients in rural areas
       through the use of telephone and video conferencing is termed:

       a.   community nursing center.
       b.   wellness program.
       c.   parish nurse program.
       d.   telehealth program.

b
Knowledge
Planning
Safety: Management
of Care

7-10   Which of the following statements is included in the Pew Health
       Professions Commission report "Healthy America?"

       a.   Maintain the current health care system.
       b.   Continue to learn.
       c.   Practice in a health care environment that supports Pew's ethical
            stand on health care.
       d.   Minimize the use of technology to control costs.

Comprehension
Planning
Safety: Management
of Care

7-11   Which of the following description exemplifies the role of the nurse when collaborating with other health care professionals?

a. Supports clients' active involvement in health care decisions.

b. Listens to each individual's views.

c. Shares personal expertise to ensure quality client care.

d. Helps clients set mutually agreed-upon goals for health care.

Knowledge
Planning
Safety: Management
of Care

7-12   Which of the following identifies key competencies necessary for collaboration?

a. negotiation, mutual respect, and trust

b. conflict management, trust, and decision making

c. communication skills, trust, and decision making

d. negotiation, conflict management, and mutual respect

Comprehension
Planning
Safety: Management
of Care

7-13   Which of the following must a nurse do to ensure continuity of care for a client?

a. Start discharge planning upon admission.

b. Include all health care team members when planning a client's care.

c. Review the final plan with the client and other family members.

d. Review the discharge goals with the physician before introducing them to the client.

Comprehension
Planning
Safety: Management
of Care

7-14   Which of the following would be *least* appropriate action when planning the discharge of a client from an acute care facility?

a. Check on the availability of family members at home to provide care or support for the client.

b. Determine the client's financial resources to purchase medication and other supplies.

c. Make the first discharge appointment with the client's primary care physician.

d. Assess the client's home environment to make sure it will ensure a healthy convalescence.

c
Application
Planning
Safety: Management
of Care

7-15   A home care referral would be appropriate for which of the following clients?

a. a 17-year-old female client recovering with a broken leg, who lives with her family

b. a 36-year-old female client recovering after surgery to remove a benign breast lump, who lives with her husband

c. a 55-year-old male recovering after four-vessel coronary artery bypass surgery, who lives alone

d. a 72-year-old female recovering from pneumonia, who lives with her daughter

a   8-1   Why is it important for a nurse to assess a client's health care beliefs?
Application
Assessment   a.   It provides the nurse with information on how much the client
Promotion: believes he can influence or control health through personal
Prevention and Early   behaviors.
Detection of Disease
                           b.   It identifies risk factors that will influence the client's locus of
                                control.

                           c.   It helps to determine the impact of stress on the client's mental and
                                physical well-being.

                           d.   It validates the other assessment data collected.

a   8-2   Following the health assessment of a client, the nurse and the client
Comprehension   summarize the information. What is the best rationale for performing
Assessment   this assessment summary?
Promotion:
Prevention and Early   a.   to allow the client to validate the information obtained by the
Detection of Disease   nurse

                           b.   to change the client's health behaviors that place the client at risk
                                for health problems

                           c.   to identify behavioral or health outcomes

                           d.   to identify barriers to behavioral change

c   8-3   In the planning stage of the nursing process, the nurse acts as a(n):
Comprehension
Planning   a.   advisor.
Safety: Management
of Care   b.   counselor.

                           c.   resource person.

                           d.   decision maker.

a   8-4   A client has identified a need to improve her nutritional status. How
Application   will goals and interventions be developed?
Planning
Promotion: a.   The client will decide the goals and interventions required to meet
Prevention and Early   her need.
Detection of Disease
                           b.   The nurse will decide the goals and interventions required to meet
                                the client's need.

                           c.   The goals and interventions developed by the nurse and client will
                                need to be acceptable to the client's doctor.

                           d.   The goals and interventions will be based on nursing priorities.

8-5 The nurse develops a written contract with a client to change the client's smoking behavior. What is the purpose of this written contract?

a. to control client behavior

b. to hold the client accountable for his behavior

c. to motivate the client to follow through with selected actions

d. to identify barriers to change

8-6 In developing a plan of behavior change for a client, it is important that a 'model' is:

a. a nurse.

b. the clients physician.

c. frequently available in the beginning.

d. a person the nurse respects.

8-7 According to Leavell and Clark, primary prevention focuses on:

a. early identification of health problems.

b. prompt nursing intervention to alleviate health problems.

c. restoration and rehabilitation to optimal functioning.

d. health promotion and protection against specific health problems.

8-8 Cognitive-perceptual factors are considered to be the primary motivational mechanisms for acquiring and maintaining health-promoting behaviors. These factors include:

a. age, sex, race, and education.

b. biological characteristics.

c. family patterns of health care and interactions with health professionals.

d. definition of health, perceived control, and perceived barriers.

8-9 During a nursing assessment, the nurse learns that the client is considering going on a weight reduction diet and has gathered information on various diets. The client verbalizes plans to begin the diet in a couple of months. What stage of health behavior change is the client in?

a. precontemplation

b. preparation

c. action

d. contemplative

c
Comprehension
Assessment
Promotion:
Prevention and Early
Detection of Disease

8-10   When a nurse assesses body composition, he is determining:

a. flexibility of the joints.

b. cardiovascular endurance.

c. ratio of body fat to muscle.

d. muscle strength.

9 HOME CARE

a
Knowledge
Assessment
Safety: Management
of Care

9-1   Home health care nursing practice differs from nursing practice in acute care settings in what way?

     a.   In home health care, nurses have a higher degree of autonomy and independence.

     b.   In home health care, the nursing process is utilized to organize care.

     c.   In home health care, clients don't require intravenous therapy.

     d.   In home health care, outcome criteria are established.

c
Comprehension
Planning
Psychosocial:
Coping and
Adaptation

9-2   A home health nurse has received a referral from a hospital for a client who requires wound care. What will be the first priority for the home health nurse?

     a.   Evaluate the client's wound.

     b.   Contact the referral source to determine the supplies needed for a home visit.

     c.   Establish rapport and trust with the client.

     d.   Contact the client's physician for instructions on wound care.

c
Knowledge
Assessment
Safety: Management
of Care

9-3   The nurse has determined that her home health client will need a special bed to ensure proper healing of the client's multiple bed sores. Which one of the following agencies would be most appropriate for the home health nurse to contact?

     a.   Department of Aging

     b.   Visiting Nurses' Association

     c.   durable medical equipment company

     d.   community health nursing agency

b
Application
Planning
Safety: Management
of Care

9-4   The home health nurse has been contacted by a family that requires nursing services to provide intravenous antibiotics therapy to one of its members. What must the home health care nurse have before she can provide services to the client?

     a.   permission from the client

     b.   a physician's order

     c.   a social worker's referral

     d.   a report on the client's homebound status

d
Application
Implementation
Safety: Management
of Care

9-5 A client with a terminal disease has been admitted to home health care for pain management. During the admission process, the client tells the nurse that outside of pain control, she does not want them to use any other medical treatments to prolong her life. The family tells the nurse that they want everything done for the client that is medically possible. The nurse's role as a client advocate is to:

a. support the family's decision.

b. convince the client to undergo recommended treatments.

c. contact the physician.

d. ensure that the client's rights and desires are upheld.

b
Application
Implementation
Safety: Management
of Care

9-6 A home health nurse has identified that a client could benefit from some assistance with his personal care. Who is responsible for providing this care?

a. the home health nurses supervised by the physician

b. the family or home health aide supervised by the home health nurse

c. the respiratory therapist supervised by the home health nurse

d. the physical therapist's aide supervised by the physical therapist

a
Application
Implementation
Safety: Safety and
Infection Control

9-7 A home health nurse suggests to a client that all throw rugs from her kitchen area should be removed. This suggestion is designed to:

a. prevent falls.

b. ensure infection control procedures are followed.

c. prevent fires.

d. promote client independence.

a
Application
Evaluation
Safety: Safety and
Infection Control

9-8 The home health nurse demonstrates how to change the client's dressing to the client's wife. Which of the following statements by the wife indicates an understanding of infection control?

a. "I should wash my hands before and after the dressing change and throw the old dressing in a plastic bag and close it."

b. "I wash my hands after I change the dressing and throw the old dressing in the trash."

c. "I put on gloves whenever I am near my husband's dressing, even when I am not changing it."

d. "I put the new dressing on, take the old one off, and wash my hands."

9-9   The home health nurse is explaining to the client's caregiver how to change the dressing on a PIC line. The caregiver asks the nurse to explain the procedure three times. When the nurse asked the caregiver to demonstrate the procedure, the caregiver states, "I can't do it now, I have to start lunch." What is the nurse's best response to this?

    a.   "I understand that this procedure may be frightening. Let me talk you through it."

    b.   "You can fix lunch later. You need to do this while I am here."

    c.   "Okay, I will do it this time, but next time you will have to do it."

    d.   "You won't do anything wrong because I have faith in you."

9-10   On the third home health visit, the nurse notices that the client's wife is withdrawn and the environment is generally not clean. The nurse notes that these may be signs of caregiver role strain. What nursing action will be most beneficial in this situation?

    a.   Sit with the wife and empathize with her.

    b.   Discuss activities that the wife could use assistance with and identify sources of help.

    c.   Perform a nursing physical assessment on the wife and report variations from normal to the physician.

    d.   Perform a nursing physical assessment on the client to ensure that he has not been abused.

b
Knowledge
Safety: Management
of Care

10-1   Nursing informatics is best defined as the science of:

    a.   delivering nursing care via computers.

    b.   supporting nursing practice with computerized systems.

    c.   storing nursing knowledge and literature on computer systems.

    d.   using electronic monitoring and charting systems.

d
Knowledge
Safety: Management
of Care

10-2   Large amounts of information are stored on computers. The volume of data is measured in:

    a.   RAM (random access memory).

    b.   mHz (megahertz).

    c.   milliseconds.

    d.   bytes.

a
Comprehension
Safety: Management
of Care

10-3   Nurses are expected to demonstrate some computer literacy. At a minimum, nurses should be able to use computers for:

    a.   word processing.

    b.   spreadsheet data entry.

    c.   statistical analysis.

    d.   database manipulation.

c
Knowledge
Safety: Management
of Care

10-4   Many hospitals communicate notices, reports, lab data, and other information via a network or local area network (LAN). Which of the following best describes a computer network?

    a.   the combination of a computer monitor, CPU, keyboard, and printer

    b.   the use of personal computers to send files from one location to another

    c.   linkages between several computers that permit sharing of data files

    d.   several personal computers using the same software

a
Knowledge
Safety: Management
of Care

10-5   Which of the following best describes the function of a Hospital Information System (HIS)?

    a.   It organizes a hospital's client and institutional databases.

    b.   It connects a hospital's personal computers to the Internet.

    c.   It provides instruction on hospital-related topics to clients.

    d.   It is a national compilation of statistics on hospital characteristics.

c
Application
Safety: Management
of Care

10-6 A nurse needs to know if there are any research studies on the optimal length of time bedridden clients can remain in one position. The electronic source most likely to provide this information for the nurse is:

a. the World Wide Web.

b. the Internet.

c. Cumulative Index to Nursing and Allied Health Literature (CINAHL).

d. computer-assisted-instruction (CAI).

b
Knowledge
Safety: Management
of Care

10-7 Computers can be used to transmit data, voice, and video across long distances. When the recipient accesses the transmission at a different time than when the person sent it, this is referred to as:

a. synchronous.

b. asynchronous.

c. random access.

d. digitized.

d
Comprehension
Safety: Management
of Care

10-8 In the United States, applicants complete the national licensure examination for registered nursing (NCLEX-RN) at a computer terminal. A computer is used because:

a. it scores the exam more accurately.

b. applicants cannot go back and change their answers.

c. more applicants can take the test at one time.

d. each applicant receives customized questions.

d
Knowledge
Safety: Management
of Care

10-9 Bedside data entry permits nurses to record client information at or near the client's location. Current research has shown conclusively that bedside data entry compared to handwritten recording is:

a. more accurate.

b. more timely.

c. more accurate and more timely.

d. not more accurate or more timely.

c
Application
Safety: Management
of Care

10-10 There are both advantages and disadvantages to computer-based patient records (CPRs). Which of the following is a significant concern about CPRs for both nurses and clients?

a. lack of standardization among systems in different health agencies

b. possibility of the computer systems malfunctioning

c. difficulty maintaining privacy and security

d. time involved in learning how to use the systems

a
Application
Safety: Management
of Care

10-11   Which of the following is an example of telemedicine or telenursing?

    a.   consulting on a client via live video 100 miles away

    b.   monitoring the EKG of a client in her room while at the nurse's station

    c.   performing surgery using robotic assistance

    d.   using a computer program to select an appropriate care plan based on the client assessment data

b
Application
Safety: Management
of Care

10-12   From the perspective of accrediting organizations, computerized systems used to manage client data and outcomes:

    a.   are discouraged until better systems become available.

    b.   must use standardized language.

    c.   should be limited to use in inpatient facilities.

    d.   are most effective in the areas of finance and budget control.

a
Application
Safety: Management
of Care

10-13   One of the uses of computers in nursing administration is for quality assurance and utilization review. One benefit of using computers for this function is the ability to:

    a.   measure achievement of desired institutional outcomes.

    b.   see if quality has been achieved.

    c.   increase accuracy in billing.

    d.   predict staffing needs.

b
Comprehension
Safety: Management
of Care

10-14   Which of the following is an example of computer use in the data collection/analysis step of the research process?

    a.   searching literature databases to identify related studies

    b.   coding data for statistical manipulation

    c.   testing prospective instruments/tools

    d.   word-processing study results for publication

b
Comprehension
Assessment
Promotion:
Prevention and Early
Detection of Disease

11-1   At the termination of an examination, the physician remarked to the client that the client exhibited no signs or symptoms of disease or illness. This client would be considered healthy by which model of health?

     a.   adaptive

     b.   clinical

     c.   role performance

     d.   eudaemonistic

c
Knowledge
Assessment
Promotion:
Prevention and Early
Detection of Disease

11-2   The actions people take to understand their health state, maintain their health, or prevent illness and injury are called:

     a.   health status.

     b.   health beliefs.

     c.   health behaviors.

     d.   health values.

b
Application
Analysis
Promotion:
Prevention and Early
Detection of Disease

11-3   A single mother of three school-age children is concerned about maintaining her present problem-free health status. Although she knows that she should exercise regularly, her job and the classes she is taking at the local community college require all of her spare time. Where is this client on Dunn's health grid?

     a.   high-level wellness in a favorable environment

     b.   emergent high-level wellness in an unfavorable environment

     c.   protected poor health in a favorable environment

     d.   poor health in an unfavorable environment

d
Knowledge
Assessment
Promotion:
Prevention and Early
Detection of Disease

11-4   Statistically, a four-year-old child is at greatest risk of dying from:

     a.   cancer.

     b.   influenza.

     c.   measles.

     d.   accidental injury.

a
Comprehension
Analysis
Promotion:
Prevention and Early
Detection of Disease

11-5   A client is considered healthy according to the eudaemonistic model of health:

     a.   when he realizes his full potential.

     b.   as long as he is able to continue working.

     c.   when he can adjust to changes in his environment.

     d.   as long as he is able to adapt to stresses.

c
Comprehension
Assessment
Promotion:
Prevention and Early
Detection of
Disease:

11-6 A 69-year-old client has a positive attitude and states that he will live to be 100 years old because he enjoys everything about his full, active life. Based on this information about the client, which variable is exerting a positive influence on his life and health?

a. age

b. culture

c. self-concept

d. standard of living

a
Application
Analysis
Promotion:
Prevention and Early
Detection of Disease

11-7 A client has been treating his severe cough and chest congestion with rest and fluids. His condition worsens and he seeks medical treatment. The physician diagnoses bacterial pneumonia. According to Smith's adaptive model, this illness is considered to be a(n):

a. failure to adapt.

b. opportunity for self-reflection.

c. alteration in body functions.

d. failure of self-actualization.

b
Comprehension
Assessment
Promotion:
Prevention and Early
Detection of Disease

11-8 A 59-year-old Latin American client noticed a lump in her breast, but she delayed seeking health treatment because from her cultural perspective, as long as one can still work, health treatment is not sought. Which of the following variables appears to be a factor in this client's health behavior?

a. demographic

b. family and cultural beliefs

c. self-concept

d. life-style choices

c
Comprehension
Analysis
Physiological:
Pharmacological and
Parenteral Therapies

11-9 Which of the following clients is expressing noncompliance?

a. the 24-year-old new mother who quits nursing her baby

b. the 45-year-old client who cannot afford to get his prescription refilled

c. the 40-year-old client who voluntarily quits taking his blood pressure medicine

d. the 18-year-old client who does not know she should take all of her antibiotics even after her symptoms are gone

b
Knowledge
Promotion:
Prevention and Early
Detection of Disease

11-10 "Illness includes all aspects of the total person, not just the disease-producing biological and genetic factors." This statement expresses a focus that has traditionally been held by:

a. medicine.

b. nursing.

c. all health care providers.

d. hospital administrators.

c
Comprehension
Assessment
Psychosocial:
Coping and
Adaptation

11-11 A 48-year-old housewife and mother of three teenage children has been hospitalized with a medical diagnosis of gallstones and is scheduled for surgery. Which effect will her hospitalization most likely to have on her family?

a. loss of privacy for the family

b. decrease in income for the family

c. alteration of family member's roles and tasks

d. loss of autonomy for the children

d
Knowledge
Implementation
Promotion:
Prevention and Early
Detection of Disease

11-12 Nurses need to model wellness behaviors because:

a. they will be respected by the medical community.

b. nurses' energy levels must be high in order to meet clients' demands.

c. the nursing profession is stressful; therefore, risk of illness is increased.

d. nurses' actions influence clients more than the information they teach.

a
Comprehension
Promotion:
Prevention and Early
Detection of Disease

11-13 What is an advantage of using the Travis Illness-Wellness Continuum as a model?

a. It can be used together with the traditional illness treatment model.

b. It emphasizes the importance of the environment on health.

c. It separates the environment into factors that lead to illness from the other factors.

d. It highlights the importance of genetic makeup and cultural influences on wellness.

b
Knowledge
Analysis
Promotion:
Prevention and Early
Detection of Disease

11-14 Which is of the following is defined as "an alteration in body functions resulting in a reduction of capacities or a shortening of the normal life span"?

a. illness

b. disease

c. acute illness

d. deviance

d
Comprehension
Analysis
Physiological:
Physiological
Adaptation

11-15 A client has chronic arthritis. After a pain-free period that lasted four weeks, he is beginning to have a great deal of pain in his hips and knees. His pain-free period is referred to as a period of:

a. deviance.

b. chronicity.

c. exacerbation.

d. remission

d
Comprehension
Assessment
Promotion:
Prevention and Early
Detection of Disease

11-16　Which statement made by a young Latin American client indicates that she believes the locus of control of her health status is external?

　　a.　"Both my mother and my grandmother are diabetic."

　　b.　"Latinos are prone to diabetes."

　　c.　"My diabetes was much better when I was pregnant."

　　d.　"My prognosis is in God's hands."

b
Application
Assessment
Promotion:
Prevention and Early
Detection of Disease

11-17　Three weeks following a heart attack, a 45-year-old football coach continues to stay at home unshaven and in his pajamas. He does not involve himself in family decisions and his family relationships have become strained. What state of Suchman's illness behavior is he demonstrating?

　　a.　denial of illness

　　b.　dependent client

　　c.　assumption of sick role

　　d.　rehabilitation

a
Analysis
Assessment
Promotion:
Prevention and Early
Detection of Disease

11-18　Under the role performance model, which of the following persons would be considered healthy?

　　a.　a nurse in renal failure who continues to work on a dialysis unit

　　b.　a concert pianist who cancels his performances to recover from surgery to his hands

　　c.　a jockey who repairs harnesses after a riding accident ended his career

　　d.　a farmer who retires because of respiratory disorders resulting from his use of pesticides

a
Application
Assessment
Promotion:
Prevention and Early
Detection of Disease

11-19　Which of the following is an illness behavior that illustrates Suchman's stage of Symptom Experiences?

　　a.　consulting with co-workers and family about symptoms

　　b.　excusing self from normal duties and expectations in order to apply home remedies to relieve symptoms

　　c.　seeking a health care professional for the diagnosis of symptoms

　　d.　becoming fearful and anxious about symptoms

c
Analysis
Assessment
Promotion:
Prevention and Early
Detection of Disease

11-20　Using the agent-host-environment model of health and illness, which of the following persons would be most prone to illness?

　　a.　a 22-year-old auto mechanic in Arizona with a mild respiratory disorder

　　b.　a 50-year-old bartender in Texas whose father is an alcoholic

　　c.　a 45-year-old air traffic controller in New York whose father is hypertensive

　　d.　an 18-year-old runner in Colorado whose mother has diabetes

d
Application
Assessment
Psychosocial:
Coping and
Adaptation

12-1   A 45-year-old client recently lost her job only a week after her husband disappeared. A nurse applying the concept of holism would consider that these events in this client's social status could cause changes in her:

     a.   emotional health, but not her spiritual health.

     b.   spiritual health, but not her physical health.

     c.   emotional health only.

     d.   emotional, physical, and spiritual health.

a
Comprehension
Promotion:
Prevention and Early
Detection of Disease

12-2   The concept of homeostasis is most like the concept of:

     a.   equilibrium.

     b.   holism.

     c.   needs.

     d.   exchange

b
Comprehension
Analysis
Promotion:
Prevention and Early
Detection of Disease

12-3   When blood volume is lost, the blood pressure falls and the heart rate increases to counteract the loss of pressure. This illustrates which aspect of the homeostatic mechanism?

     a.   decompensation

     b.   compensation

     c.   self-regulation

     d.   equilibrium

a
Comprehension
Assessment
Psychosocial:
Coping and
Adaptation

12-4   For which of the following persons is psychologic homeostasis threatened?

     a.   an adult who has been homeless and hungry for several periods during his life and has recently become homeless again

     b.   an adolescent who receives kind but firm and consistent discipline

     c.   a child who has adults who model the customs and values of their society and reward the child for similar behavior

     d.   an adult who is presently frustrated in his efforts to make changes in his work environment, but mostly has satisfying experiences throughout his life

c
Comprehension
Assessment
Psychosocial:
Coping and
Adaptation

12-5   According to Maslow, once a need is completely met, the individual:

     a.   is considered to be self-actualized.

     b.   has achieved total health.

     c.   is no longer aware of the need.

     d.   focuses upon gaining knowledge.

a
Knowledge
Psychosocial:
Coping and
Adaptation

12-6 In Maslow's hierarchy of needs, which category of needs must be met before a person can focus upon safety and security needs?

a. physiologic
b. self-esteem
c. love and belonging
d. self-actualization

d
Knowledge
Assessment
Psychosocial:
Coping and
Adaptation

12-7 In Maslow's hierarchy of needs, the self-actualized person:

a. is other-directed.
b. possesses above-normal intelligence.
c. has a future-time orientation.
d. has realized his/her full potential.

c
Comprehension
Analysis
Psychosocial:
Coping and
Adaptation

12-8 Which of the following is an example of a deferred need?

a. thinking about food, which stimulates hunger and the need for food
b. having a cocktail to meet the need for relaxation
c. withdrawing from school until recovery from an illness is complete
d. a respiratory obstruction creates a need for oxygen, which alters security needs

b
Comprehension
Promotion:
Prevention and Early
Detection of Disease

12-9 Von Bertalanffy's general systems theory is useful because it:

a. is specifically concerned with health care.
b. is a universal theory; it can be applied to many fields of study.
c. has replaced the germ theory of disease.
d. was developed by a nursing theorist especially to help nurses meet clients' psychosocial needs.

a
Knowledge
Promotion: Growth
and Development
Through the Life
Span

12-10 *Family-centered nursing care* can be defined as nursing that is concerned with:

a. the health of both the family unit and the individual members.
b. maintaining and strengthening the family.
c. providing health care during the period of pregnancy and birth.
d. providing care in the home with the help of the family members.

c
Knowledge
Analysis
Psychosocial:
Coping and
Adaptation

12-11 After the death of her husband, a 67-year-old client goes to live with her daughter, son-in law, and two grandchildren. With this addition, the family unit has changed from a(n):

a. extended family to a cohabiting family.
b. blended family to a nuclear family.
c. nuclear family to an extended family.
d. cohabiting family to a nuclear family.

a
Comprehension
Assessment
Promotion: Growth
and Development
Through the Life
Span

12-12   What is a basic role of the family?

     a.   to protect and socialize its members

     b.   to produce goods necessary for survival

     c.   to establish a primary place of residence

     d.   to produce offspring to replenish society

a
Application
Analysis
Promotion: Growth
and Development
Through the Life
Span

12-13   Which of the following family structures would fit the current definition of a *traditional family*?

     a.   Father provides income. Mother provides care of home and children.

     b.   Father and mother provide income and share responsibility for household chores and child care.

     c.   Father and mother provide income. Mother responsible for household duties and child care.

     d.   Mother provides income. Father provides care of home and children.

d
Knowledge
Analysis
Promotion: Growth
and Development
Through the Life
Span

12-14   A nurse could most logically infer that a 'latch key kid' is a member of a:

     a.   blended family.

     b.   lesbian family.

     c.   traditional family.

     d.   two-career family.

c
Knowledge
Assessment
Promotion: Growth
and Development
Through the Life
Span

12-15   The type of family unit that presents the highest risk for fatigue, role overload, poverty, and depression is the:

     a.   blended family.

     b.   gay or lesbian family.

     c.   single-parent family.

     d.   two-career family.

12-16   A major sociologic risk factor for developing health problems is:

     a.   poverty.

     b.   adolescent mothers.

     c.   lack of daily exercise.

     d.   genetic predisposition to disease.

12-17   The nursing diagnosis defined by the North American Nursing Diagnosis Association as "the state in which a normally supportive family experiences a stressor that affects its functioning" refers to:

     a.   Ineffective Family Coping, Disabling.

     b.   Ineffective Family Coping, Compromised.

     c.   Altered Family Processes.

     d.   Family Coping: Potential for Growth.

c
Analysis
Assessment
Psychosocial:
Coping and
Adaptation

12-18 Which statement best illustrates the sense of disorganization experienced by a family member at the death of a close relative?

a. "Mom is at rest now. She is not hurting anymore."

b. "Dad still had so much to offer. He should not have died so young."

c. "Nothing will ever be the same now that Mom is gone."

d. "Mom is with God and all her family that has gone on before her."

d
Comprehension
Analysis
Promotion: Growth
and Development
Through the Life
Span

12-19 Which of the following is an example of a *community of interest*?

a. city with an elected mayor

b. traditional family

c. country with a complex political system

d. group protesting the use of animals for medical research

b
Comprehension
Assessment
Promotion:
Prevention and Early
Detection of Disease

12-20 In order to individualize care, it is most important that the nurse:

a. be knowledgeable about the pathophysiology of the client's disease.

b. determine how the client perceives and interprets what is happening to him.

c. support the client's homeostatic mechanisms.

d. have family members take part in the client's care.

d
Analysis
Assessment
Psychosocial:
Coping and
Adaptation

12-21 Using Maslow's framework, which statement characterizes a self-actualized person?

a. "I have a driving need to change the world."

b. "I don't want any changes made from the way it has always been."

c. "I will look like a fool if I admit that my idea is not working."

d. "I have listened to everyone, but I still have to do what I think is right."

b
Knowledge
Assessment
Psychosocial:
Coping and
Adaptation

12-22 Which assessment would give the nurse the most insight into a family's values?

a. age and sex of the family members

b. religious and cultural practices

c. ability to meet financial needs

d. how the household tasks are distributed

c
Comprehension
Assessment
Psychosocial:
Coping and
Adaptation

12-23   Which of the following illnesses would probably have the greatest impact on a family?

a.   a serious illness from which the family member recovers quickly

b.   an acute illness that leaves no permanent disability on the family member

c.   a long-term illness with progressively disabling effects on the family member

d.   a permanent illness that has minor effects on the family member

d
Knowledge
Analysis
Promotion: Growth
and Development
Through the Life
Span

12-24   Which of the following is a characteristic of a healthy community?

a.   allows groups in the community to solve disputes among themselves in their own way

b.   has a smoothly functioning government that requires minimal citizen participation

c.   socially controls subgroups so that they do not influence community decisions

d.   makes system resources available to all members of the community

a
Knowledge
Promotion: Growth
and Development
Through the Life
Span

13-1 Culture is best defined as the:

a. traditions, values, and norms transmitted from generation to generation.

b. classification of people according to shared biologic characteristics.

c. group religious or racial characteristics that set it apart from the larger society of which it is a part.

d. assumption of attitudes, values, and beliefs of the dominant society.

c
Knowledge
Analysis
Psychosocial:
Coping and
Adaptation

13-2 Belief that one's culture is superior to all others is called:

a. discrimination.

b. stereotyping.

c. ethnocentrism.

d. racism.

c
Knowledge
Psychosocial:
Coping and
Adaptation

13-3 Changing cultural traditions due to environmental differences reflects which of the following characteristics of culture?

a. learned

b. social

c. adaptive

d. ideational

d
Application
Analysis
Promotion: Growth
and Development
Through the Life
Span

13-4 A 21-year-old Mexican American client has just delivered her first baby. Based on the nurse's past experience with a Mexican-American family, the nurse assumes that family members will gather to care for the mother and infant. This is an example of:

a. discrimination.

b. ethnocentrism.

c. racism.

d. stereotyping.

a
Application
Analysis
Psychosocial:
Coping and
Adaptation

13-5 The first generation of a Chinese family used herbal remedies to treat their illnesses. However, members of the third North American generation obtain their health care from a medical doctor, the same as most North Americans. This is an example of:

a. assimilation.

b. ethnocentrism.

c. culture shock.

d. cultural competence.

d
Application
Assessment
Promotion: Growth
and Development
Through the Life
Span

13-6   A young Latin American client who has just had a baby tells the nurse
        that she will breastfeed her baby. She says, "My husband thinks all
        mothers should breastfeed." The client's decision reflects that the
        traditional Mexican American culture is:

        a. bicultural.

        b. ideational.

        c. matriarchal.

        d. patriarchal.

c
Application
Implementation
Promotion: Growth
and Development
Through the Life
Span

13-7   A Mexican American client who has just had a baby tells the nurse that
        she will breastfeed her baby. She says, "My husband thinks all mothers
        should breastfeed." The European American nurse suggests to the client
        that she should breastfeed only if *she* wants to and not because of her
        husband's influence. The nurse's suggestion reflects:

        a. assimilation.

        b. biculturalism.

        c. ethnocentrism.

        d. stereotyping.

d
Comprehension
Analysis
Psychosocial:
Coping and
Adaptation

13-8   A Jewish client asks the nurse, "Why am I sick? I haven't committed any
        sins." This statement reflects a belief that illness is:

        a. something that cannot be prevented.

        b. disharmony with the forces of nature.

        c. an imbalance in life forces.

        d. a punishment from God.

d
Comprehension
Assessment
Psychosocial:
Coping and
Adaptation

13-9   During the admission interview, a Native American client responds to
        direct questions, but does not volunteer any information or elaborate in
        response to open-ended questions. His reluctance to talk may be related
        to a cultural belief that:

        a. hospitalization is an invasion of privacy.

        b. health care is not harmonious with nature.

        c. the female role is one of subservience to the male.

        d. silence shows respect and is valuable in understanding another's
            needs.

b
Application
Implementation
Psychosocial:
Coping and
Adaptation

13-10   A Native American client admitted to the hospital for surgery asks if his
        medicine man can perform a 30-minute healing ceremony prior to
        surgery. The nurse should:

        a. tell him that such rituals are not part of the preoperative preparation

        b. provide the space and privacy for the ceremony.

        c. explain that in modern health care there is no need for medicine men.

        d. request the hospital chaplain to pray with the client.

d
Application
Implementation
Safety: Management
of Care

13-11   A 50-year-old recent immigrant from Poland who speaks no English, has been hospitalized for severe pelvic inflammatory disease. Which bilingual person should be asked to interpret for this client?

a. the client's 14-year-old daughter

b. the client's husband

c. a 45-year-old male respiratory therapist

d. a 34-year-old female bookkeeper in the hospital

c
Knowledge
Promotion:
Prevention and Early
Detection of Disease

13-12   Chinese folk medicine proposes that the universe and health are regulated by two forces:

a. wet and dry.

b. good and bad.

c. yin and yang.

d. harmony and nature.

a
Knowledge
Assessment
Psychosocial:
Coping and
Adaptation

13-13   The feelings experienced by individuals when they enter an unfamiliar environment such as the hospital are called:

a. culture shock.

b. acculturation.

c. discrimination.

d. assimilation.

b
Application
Analysis
Psychosocial:
Coping and
Adaptation

13-14   The nurse in the community health clinic has noticed that many Latin American and African American clients arrive as much as one or two hours late for their appointments. What cultural interpretation would explain this pattern?

a. rejection of the Protestant work ethic

b. relaxed orientation to time

c. low value on health maintenance

d. resistance to community health care

d
Application
Analysis
Promotion:
Prevention and Early
Detection of Disease

13-15   A 60-year-old African American female client does not maintain direct eye contact with the nurse during the intake interview in the health clinic. The nurse should:

a. intensify his own eye contact with the client.

b. request the client to look at him when responding to questions.

c. position himself to facilitate eye contact with the client.

d. model his own eye contact to be similar to the client's.

c
Application
Evaluation
Promotion:
Prevention and Early
Detection of Disease

13-16   When caring for a client from a different culture who does not speak the nurse's language, a culturally sensitive nurse should:

a.   make liberal use of touch to communicate with the client.

b.   interpret smiling and nodding to mean that the client understands what the nurse has said.

c.   observe the client's response to touch and only use touch that she is certain is acceptable to the client.

d.   interpret smiling and nodding to mean that the client likes the nurse and agrees with what she is saying.

a
Comprehension
Assessment
Promotion:
Prevention and Early
Detection of Disease

13-17   For which client would the nurse probably have most difficulty 'reading' facial expressions? One who has recently moved to North America from:

a.   England.

b.   Puerto Rico.

c.   Italy.

d.   Mexico.

a
Application
Analysis
Safety: Management
of Care

13-18   For which of the following clients should a male nurse or physician probably do the discharge teaching and planning?

a.   Middle Eastern male client

b.   Japanese male client

c.   African American female client

d.   Latin American female client

a
Application
Implementation
Promotion: Growth
and Development
Through the Life
Span

13-19   A nurse has insisted that a family not tape a coin to their newborn infant's umbilicus, despite their cultural beliefs and over their protests. The family will most likely react with:

a.   distrust.

b.   respect.

c.   confidence.

d.   ridicule.

b
Knowledge
Assessment
Psychosocial:
Coping and
Adaptation

13-20   Which assessment would give the nurse the most insight into a family's values?

a.   age and sex of the family members

b.   their religious and cultural practices

c.   ability to meet financial needs

d.   how the household tasks are distributed

13-21 A 45-year-old Chinese woman resists following a prescribed bland diet that recommends dishes using potatoes and turkey. Which intervention by the nurse would most likely encourage compliance?

    a. Assure client that the meals on the prescribed diet are wholesome and nutritious.

    b. Help client identify the foods on the bland diet as a treatment for her illness.

    c. Write out complex menus to meet nutritional needs using potatoes and turkey.

    d. Negotiate with the client to substitute fish and rice for potatoes and turkey.

13-22 A client remarks that he only buys American cars because American cars are better made than any European or Asian cars. This is an example of:

    a. stereotyping.

    b. prejudice.

    c. racism.

    d. ethnorelativity.

14 SPIRITUALITY

d
Knowledge
Assessment
Psychosocial:
Coping and
Adaptation

14-1 In Murray and Zentner's framework, spirituality focuses on:

    a. purpose and meaning in life.

    b. one's relationship with God.

    c. one's relationship with self and others.

    d. harmony with the universe.

a
Knowledge
Assessment
Psychosocial:
Coping and
Adaptation

14-2 *Religion* is best defined as:

    a. an organized system of worship.

    b. a belief in some higher power.

    c. harmony with the universe.

    d. a focus on the purpose and meaning in life.

d
Knowledge
Assessment
Psychosocial:
Coping and
Adaptation

14-3 *Spirituality* may be defined as:

    a. an organized system of worship.

    b. the acceptance of specific rituals.

    c. being committed to something.

    d. a belief in or relationship with some higher power.

a
Comprehension
Analysis
Psychosocial:
Coping and
Adaptation

14-4 A client says, "I'm not saying that God doesn't exist. I'm saying that no one has proven that God exists." This client could be said to be:

    a. agnostic.

    b. atheistic.

    c. monotheistic.

    d. polytheistic.

d
Knowledge
Implementation
Safety: Management
of care

14-5 Meeting the spiritual needs of clients and their families is part of the function of:

    a. the nursing staff.

    b. the hospital clergy.

    c. the clients' specific religious group.

    d. caregivers and the clients' usual religious group.

a
Knowledge
Assessment
Psychosocial:
Coping and
Adaptation

14-6 A person who denies the existence of God or a supreme being is called a(n):

    a. atheist.

    b. agnostic.

    c. theist.

    d. monotheist.

b
Knowledge
Assessment
Psychosocial:
Coping and
Adaptation

14-7   The belief that parents, like God, are omnipotent, is characteristic of which spiritual developmental stage?

a.   infants and toddlers

b.   preschoolers

c.   school-age children

d.   young adults

a
Knowledge
Planning
Psychosocial:
Coping and
Adaptation

14-8   Individuals of the Islamic religion have some dietary restrictions. For example, they must avoid:

a.   pork and alcohol.

b.   fish and caffeine.

c.   veal and cow's milk.

d.   beef and citrus.

b
Comprehension
Analysis
Psychosocial:
Coping and
Adaptation

14-9   An elderly client who is a Seventh Day Adventist is scheduled to undergo a right total hip replacement for a fracture she sustained at the neck of the femur. What effect could her religion have on her treatment?

a.   Because she does not eat meat, it will be difficult to supply her with the protein her body needs for healing.

b.   If a blood transfusion is needed, she will probably refuse it because her religious group is opposed to blood transfusions.

c.   She must receive holy communion before surgery, which may delay the surgery.

d.   Any removed body parts or tissue must be buried.

a
Comprehension
Implementation
Psychosocial:
Coping and
Adaptation

14-10 A young Roman Catholic female client just gave birth to a premature baby with very serious respiratory difficulties. It is important to know that based on the young mother's religion, she may:

a.   want the infant to be baptized because its life is in danger.

b.   be opposed to blood transfusions.

c.   want to receive Holy Communion as soon as possible.

d.   require that removed body part or tissues (such as the placenta) be buried.

a
Application
Planning
Psychosocial:
Coping and
Adaptation

14-11 A client with terminal cancer expresses extreme anger about an unsolicited visit by the hospital chaplain. He furiously states that he wants nothing to do with a god who has allowed him to suffer. In planning interventions to help this client cope effectively with spiritual distress, an appropriate outcome criterion would be that he:

a. verbalize relief of anger toward the transcendent being, self, and others.

b. stop complaining about the hospital chaplain's visits.

c. is involved in diversional activities that prevent him from dwelling on his problem.

d. experience conversion and a sense of forgiveness.

d
Application
Assessment
Psychosocial:
Coping and
Adaptation

14-12 To help alleviate spiritual distress effectively, the nurse must:

a. learn as much as possible about the practices of the client's religious group.

b. offer to pray with the client.

c. recognize that "No religious affiliation" on the client's record indicates that the client is an agnostic and has no spiritual needs.

d. find out what the client perceives his/her spiritual needs to be.

d
Comprehension
Assessment
Psychosocial:
Coping and
Adaptation

14-13 According to Fowler, faith is:

a. dependent on religious development.

b. proven through logical thought processes.

c. perceiving realistic expectations and goals

d. present in both religious and nonreligious people.

d
Comprehension
Assessment
Psychosocial:
Coping and
Adaptation

14-14 Using the framework of Westerhoff's four stages of faith, a person would be most likely to stand up for his or her beliefs against the nurturing community as a:

a. preschooler in the experience faith stage.

b. late adolescent in the affiliative faith stage.

c. young adult in the searching faith stage.

d. middle-aged or older adult in the owned faith stage.

a
Comprehension
Implementation
Psychosocial:
Coping and
Adaptation

14-15 A Muslim client is dying. Because the nurse has discussed death with the family, she knows that:

a. a Muslim must perform ritual cleansing and preparation of the body for burial.

b. the chaplain should be called to anoint the body.

c. if a religious leader is not available, she should baptize the client before he dies.

d. the family will not want to touch the body or remain in the room after the client dies.

14-16   In which religion is infant baptism a practice?

a. Baha'i

b. Buddhism

c. Judaism

d. Roman Catholicism

14-17 Which religion prohibits removal of body hair?

a. Baha'i

b. Buddhism

c. Islam

d. Sikhism

14-18 For which clients should the nurse seriously consider that the statement "I'm sick because God is punishing me" may be a normal finding rather than a defining characteristic for the NANDA diagnosis of Spiritual Distress?

a. Buddhist
b. Muslim
c. Orthodox Jew
d. Hindu

14-19 A nurse midwife is attending at the home birth of a Roman Catholic child who is born with life-threatening disorders. Death appears imminent. The distraught family becomes very emotional and requests that the nurse baptize the infant. The most appropriate response by the nurse would be:

a. "I am not an ordained minister and have no authority to do so."

b. "I will ask the Supreme Being's love and protection for this new life."

c. "I am not Catholic. Any of you can perform a baptism."

d. "I cannot baptize your baby, but I will say a prayer to relieve your stress."

14-20 When an elderly Muslim client asks the nurse, "Which direction is east?," the nurse recognizes this request may be an indication the client:

a. believes that his death is near.

b. must pray at the break of dawn.

c. must bathe immediately after sunrise.

d. believes the rising sun has healing power.

d
Application
Planning
Psychosocial:
Coping and
Adaptation

14-21 Which dietary adjustment would support a hospitalized Muslim's spiritual wellness during Ramadan?

a. arranging for only one large meal to be served in the middle of the day

b. including whole grain foods and fresh fruit with each meal

c. providing herbal teas and unleavened bread before each meal

d. requesting that meals be served before dawn and after sunset

d
Analysis
Intervention
Psychosocial:
Coping and
Adaptation

14-22 A blind Jewish client who speaks and understands very little English has asked to hear the 'holy words' prior to his surgery. The most appropriate nursing intervention would be to request:

a. the hospital chaplain to read passages from the Old Testament.

b. a member of the client's family to read from the Koran.

c. a rabbi to read from the Veda.

d. the Yiddish translator to read from the Torah.

c
Application
Intervention
Psychosocial:
Coping and
Adaptation

14-23 A 22-year-old client who is in the advanced stages of AIDS says to his primary nurse, "I know that I am not going to get better. I think I would like to pray, but I do not know how. I don't even know to whom." The most supportive response the nurse could make at this time would be:

a. "It is frightening to be facing the end of your life. I will pray for you."

b. "I will call the chaplain to speak with you about this."

c. "What do you want to say in your prayer?"

d. "Many people your age have been alienated by religion."

c
Comprehension
Implementation
Psychosocial:
Coping and
Adaptation

15-1   A nurse is caring for a 16-year-old client who has had a total hysterectomy (removal of uterus, ovaries and tubes) would demonstrate a holistic approach by:

a. focusing on the drastic changes in the menstrual cycle.

b. teaching the importance and long-term benefits of hormone replacement.

c. considering how the loss of the uterus would affect the client's body, mind and spirit.

d. assisting client to plan for alternatives to natural parenthood.

d
Knowledge
Promotion:
Prevention and Early
Detection of Disease

15-2   Holistic health belief is based on the:

a. linear, logical processes of the left brain.

b. intuitive, creative processes of the right brain.

c. holiness of the body as a spiritual entity.

d. balance and harmony of the whole person.

c
Knowledge
Promotion:
Prevention and Early
Detection of Disease

15-3   Using Barbara Dossey's eras of medicine model, which approach would be considered an Era II intervention?

a. radiation

b. intercessory prayer

c. biofeedback

d. shamanic healing

c
Knowledge
Physiological:
Physiological
Adaptation

15-4   The concept of *curing* differs from the concept of *healing* in that curing focuses on:

a. active client participation.

b. client's interpretation and reaction to the pathophysiology.

c. the response of the limbic-hypothalamic system.

d. use of technology and analysis to correct pathophysiology.

a
Knowledge
Implementation
Promotion:
Prevention and Early
Detection of Disease

15-5   Which of the following best describes the body-mind healing process of *information transduction*?

a. conversion of information from one form to another

b. passing of information from one source to another

c. translating feelings into information

d. understanding how several pieces of information are related

a
Application
Implementation
Psychosocial:
Coping and
Adaptation

15-6   A client with a broken leg expresses dissatisfaction with the generalized healing imagery he is using. The nurse assists him to use end-stage imagery instead. The change in imagery would be from an image of:

   a.   being bathed in warm sunlight to an image of running on a beach.

   b.   bone cells repairing the break in the leg to an image of an angel's hands soothing the discomfort.

   c.   the break in the bone looking like jagged glass to an image of a warm white light filling the leg.

   d.   broken bone becoming smooth and solid like marble to an image of a dog chewing up the bone in the leg.

c
Knowledge
Implementation
Physiological: Basic
Care and Comfort

15-7   Effective touch therapies such as massage, accupressure, and foot reflexology are designed to stimulate a therapeutic response from the parasympathetic branch of the autonomic nervous system; for example, a(n):

   a.   increase in heart rate.

   b.   rise in blood pressure.

   c.   ease in breathing.

   d.   slowing of peristalsis.

a
Application
Implementation
Physiological: Basic
Care and Comfort

15-8   When the nurse suggests music therapy for pain control, the client replies, "I can't carry a tune in a bucket." The nurse should clarify that the technique of music therapy can:

   a.   be in the form of dancing, clapping or simply listening to music.

   b.   improve his musical ability.

   c.   can put him in touch with himself if classical music is used

   d.   be used only used at bedtime.

b
Application
Planning
Psychosocial:
Coping and
Adaptation

15-9   A nurse wants to incorporate humor in her nursing care on a surgery unit. Which of the following strategies would be the most effective?

   a.   Doing an imitation of a confused surgeon for a surgical client.

   b.   Collecting cartoons related to surgery and surgical clients.

   c.   Telling surgical jokes to a client just prior to surgery.

   d.   Tuning the client's TV to shows the nurse perceives as humorous.

a
Comprehension
Promotion:
Prevention and Early
Detection of Disease

15-10 Meditation and yoga are similar in that they both utilize:

a. structured movements and body positions.

b. rapid and forceful breathing to increase the oxygen level in the cells.

c. concentration on all things in the immediate area to enhance integration with nature.

d. a flexible schedule as to time of day and length of time for the therapy.

c
Application
Implementation
Promotion:
Prevention and Early
Detection of Disease

15-11 The nurse should caution a client who plans to use essential oils for aromatherapy to:

a. test for possible allergies by putting one drop of oil in the eye.

b. let the oils be warmed by direct sunlight to enhance the aroma.

c. use the oils only on the face and neck if pregnant.

d. be aware that the production of such oils is not regulated.

b
Knowledge
Implementation
Physiological: Basic
Care and Comfort

15-12 The nurse uses a technique of unruffling to:

a. assist the client to sleep.

b. mobilize congested energy fields.

c. distract the client from the health problem.

d. hypnotize the client.

c
Knowledge
Implementation
Physiological: Basic
Care and Comfort

15-13 The nurse using therapeutic touch as a holistic therapy believes that therapeutic effects are transferred from the nurse to the client through special channels called chakras located in the:

a. abdomen.

b. head.

c. thorax.

d. feet and hands.

c
Knowledge
Promotion:
Prevention and Early
Detection of Disease

15-14 The theoretical construct that "the cure of the disease lies within the disease itself" is the basis of:

a. naturapathy.

b. homeopathy.

c. acupuncture.

d. chiropractic practice.

c
Knowledge
Safety: Management
of Care

15-15 The Dietary Supplement Health and Education Act of 1994 provided that all herbs:

a. must be labeled as to their probable effects on the body functions.

b. must meet the FDA standard.

c. if labeled, must have the disclaimer the FDA has not reviewed the herb.

d. that are sold as finely ground products must be 100% pure herb.

b
Application
Evaluation
Physiological: Basic
Care and Comfort

15-16 The nurse recognizes a Knowledge Deficit related to hypnosis as a holistic therapy exists when the client says:

a. "Hypnosis can help me stop smoking."

b. "I may do something immoral while under hypnosis."

c. "Perception of pain can be reduced by hypnosis."

d. "Endorphins can be released through hypnosis."

a
Comprehension
Safety: Management
of Care

16-1   The nursing process and the scientific method are both systematic approaches to problem solving. The major difference between the two is that the:

     a.   scientific method is more useful in a controlled environment, such as a laboratory, than in a client care setting.

     b.   complexity of the scientific method allows the nurse to solve multiple problems rather than the individual problems studied by the nursing process.

     c.   nursing process is better adapted to the scientific control of the hospital rather than that of the laboratory.

     d.   nursing process, unlike the scientific method, formulates a hypothesis to test the stated problem.

a
Knowledge
Safety: Management
of Care

16-2   Critical thinking can best be described as:

     a.   a conscious examination of one's thinking processes.

     b.   a problem-solving process.

     c.   creativity.

     d.   the scientific method.

b
Application
Implementation
Physiological:
Pharmacological and
Parenteral Therapies

16-3   When a two-year-old client resists taking a liquid medication that is essential to her treatment, the nurse demonstrates critical thinking by:

     a.   omitting this dose of medication and waiting until the child is more cooperative.

     b.   diluting the medication with a carbonated beverage and offering it as 'sparkle juice'.

     c.   asking the head nurse about how to approach the situation.

     d.   notifying the physician that she has been unable to give the medication.

C
Application
Implementation
Safety: Safety and
Infection Control

16-4   When a new policy of restraining all four extremities of children under two years of age during IV therapy is introduced to the pediatric department, a nurse exhibits healthy skepticism by:

     a.   verbally attacking the new policy immediately.

     b.   disregarding the new policy and continuing to use only minimal restraint.

     c.   asking for the rationale behind the policy.

     d.   obeying the policy, but continuing complaining to co-workers about it.

d
Knowledge
Safety: Management
of Care

16-5 Critical thinking consists of:

a. a person's fund of knowledge.

b. the cognitive processes of the mind.

c. mental attitudes and feelings.

d. both attitudes and cognitive processes.

a
Application
Implementation
Safety: Management
of Care

16-6 The head nurse recognizes a critical thinking attitude in a new graduate when the graduate:

a. admits he does not know how to do a procedure and requests help.

b. makes his point with clever and persuasive remarks to win an argument.

c. accepts without question the values acquired in nursing school.

d. finds a quick and easy answer, even to complex questions.

b
Application
Assessment
Safety: Management
of Care

16-7 After speaking with her client, a nursing student thinks, "I don't know why, but I have the strongest feeling there is something important she is not telling me. She seems afraid to talk about it." What should the student do?

a. Chart that the client is afraid to talk about something.

b. Ask the nursing instructor to advise her about validating this feeling.

c. Trust her intuition and inform the head nurse or the physician.

d. Write on the care plan so that other nurses will try to get the data from the client.

c
Knowledge
Safety: Management
of Care

16-8 In which type of problem solving does the nurse generate hypotheses very early in the process?

a. intuitive problem solving

b. trial-and-error

c. scientific method

d. modified scientific method

d
Application
Assessment
Promotion:
Prevention and Early
Detection of Disease

16-9 A nurse knows that the nursing diagnosis of Impaired Skin Integrity involves disruption of the skin surface that can be related to physical immobility, altered nutritional state, or altered circulation. As a result, she makes sure to examine the skin of a very thin, completely paralyzed client for redness and other signs of impending disruption or breakdown. What kind of reasoning is this nurse using?

a. intuitive

b. trial-and-error

c. inductive

d. deductive

b
Comprehension
Safety: Management
of Care

16-10 How is decision making related to the nursing process?

a. They are not related. They are separate processes.

b. Decisions are required in each step of the nursing process.

c. The steps in both processes are the same, except for diagnosing.

d. Both processes require intuition.

a
Application
Analysis
Psychosocial:
Coping and
Adaptation

16-11 The nurse notes that her client is passive, shows no emotion, will make no eye contact, often sighs, and says such things as "I can't" or "It doesn't matter." The nurse believes these cues are related and may indicate a nursing diagnosis of Hopelessness. What kind of reasoning is the nurse using?

a. inductive

b. deductive

c. trial-and-error

d. intuitive

c
Application
Planning
Physiological: Basic
Care and Comfort

16-12 After designing an approach for a client who has been refusing to go to physical therapy, a nurse anticipates the problems that might occur and plans preventative measures to solve them. In the decision-making process this is called:

a. setting the criteria.

b. identifying the purpose.

c. troubleshooting.

d. evaluating the action.

a
Comprehension
Assessment
Safety: Management
of Care

16-13 According to Strader, the preparation stage of the creative process is most like which step of the nursing process?

a. assessing

b. planning

c. implementing

d. evaluating

d
Comprehension
Evaluation
Safety: Management
of Care

16-14 Which of Strader's four stages of the creative process is most like the evaluating step in the nursing process?

a. preparation

b. incubation

c. insight

d. verification

b
Comprehension
Safety: Management
of Care

16-15   Creative thinking as a problem-solving technique:

a.   is completely intuitive.

b.   requires knowledge of the problem.

c.   considers only the solutions most likely to work.

d.   uses conscious rather than unconscious processes.

b
Knowledge
Analysis
Safety: Management
of Care

16-16   In which step of the nursing process does the nurse make inferences about patterns of client data?

a.   assessing

b.   diagnosing

c.   planning

d.   implementing

d
Knowledge
Implementation
Safety: Management
of Care

16-17   Which step of the nursing process is most like the critical thinking skill of hypothesis testing?

a.   assessing

b.   diagnosing

c.   planning

d.   implementing

a
Knowledge
Safety: Management
of Care

16-18   What is the first step of the research process (scientific method)?

a.   stating a research question that specifies the intent of the study

b.   reviewing the related literature

c.   formulating hypotheses and defining variables

d.   selecting the population to be studied

A
Comprehension
Implementation
Safety: Management
of Care

16-19   A nurse who randomly tries a number of different methods to relieve a client's pain until one method is successful is using which problem-solving approach?

a.   trial-and-error

b.   intuition

c.   scientific method

d.   experimentation

c
Application
Safety: Management
of Care

16-20   Which of the following describes inductive research?

a.   A hypothesis is proposed and then research is conducted.

b.   A hypothesis is developed after research has been conducted.

c.   A theory is developed from the research findings.

d.   A theory is identified and then research is conducted.

a
Comprehension
Promotion:
Prevention and Early
Detection of Disease

17-1   The nursing process is a dynamic process. This means that it:

a. is ever changing in response to the client's needs.

b. conveys the force or power of the health team.

c. allows the client to achieve new goals each day.

d. provides solutions for client problems.

b
Knowledge
Promotion:
Prevention and Early
Detection of Disease

17-2   The nursing process components may overlap in practice. However, which of the following is the order in which they generally occur?

a. assessing, planning, diagnosing, evaluating, implementing

b. assessing, diagnosing, planning, implementing, evaluating

c. planning, assessing, diagnosing, implementing, evaluating

d. diagnosing, implementing, evaluating, assessing, planning

a
Application
Assessment
Physiological:
Physiological
Adaptation

17-3   A client comes to the clinic with vomiting and dehydration. The nurse takes his vital signs. This is an example of:

a. assessing.

b. diagnosing.

c. planning.

d. implementing.

c
Comprehension
Planning
Promotion:
Prevention and Early
Detection of Disease

17-4   In which step of the nursing process does the nurse work with the client to establish goals and desired outcomes?

a. assessing

b. diagnosing

c. planning

d   evaluating

b
Knowledge
Analysis/Diagnosis
Promotion:
Prevention and Early
Detection of Disease

17-5   In which step of the nursing process does the nurse identify actual and potential health problems?

a. assessing

b. diagnosing

c. implementing

d. evaluating

d
Comprehension
Promotion:
Prevention and Early
Detection of Disease

17-6   Which of the following best describes the nursing process?

a. It is a solution to all client problems.

b. It is useful mainly in the hospital setting.

c. It is linear in nature, progressing in separate, unrelated steps.

d. It is a systematic, problem-solving approach to client care.

c
Application
Implementation
Physiological:
Pharmacological and
Parenteral Therapies

17-7   A nurse has administered a medication to relieve a client's nausea. Which component of the nursing process does this illustrate?

a.   assessing

b.   diagnosing

c.   implementing

d.   evaluating

d
Application
Evaluation
Physiological:
Pharmacological and
Parenteral Therapies

17-8   Twenty minutes after administering an anti-nausea medication to the client, the nurse returns to ask him if he is feeling better. The nurse is:

a.   diagnosing.

b.   planning.

c.   implementing.

d.   evaluating.

b
Application
Planning
Physiological:
Pharmacological and
Parenteral Therapies

17-9   The nurse writes the following desired outcome, "Nausea will be relieved within 20 to 40 minutes following administration of Tigan (trimethobenzamide hydrochloride)." This is an example of:

a.   assessing.

b.   planning.

c.   implementing.

d.   evaluating.

d
Knowledge
Promotion:
Prevention and Early
Detection of Disease

17-10   What are the origins of the term *nursing process*?

a.   It originated with Florence Nightingale.

b.   It has been in use only since the early 1980s.

c.   It was initiated by the American Nurses Association in 1973.

d.   It was first used by Lydia Hall in 1955.

a
Knowledge
Planning
Promotion:
Prevention and Early
Detection of Disease

17-11   What is the 'product' of the planning step of the nursing process?

a.   nursing care plan

b.   nursing diagnosis

c.   note in the client's record

d.   nursing history

b
Comprehension
Promotion:
Prevention and Early
Detection of Disease

17-12   Which of the following best describes how the nursing process differs from the medical process?

a.   The nursing process requires interpersonal, technical, and intellectual skills.

b.   The nursing process focuses on client responses to illness.

c.   The nursing process focuses on identifying the client's disease process.

d.   The nursing process is not limited to use with hospitalized clients.

c
Comprehension
Safety: Management
of Care

17-13 Which of the following provides the basic framework for nurses' accountability to their clients?

a. nursing theory

b. hospital policy

c. the nursing process

d. medical orders

d
Comprehension
Safety: Management
of Care

17-14 The most important benefit of the nursing process for clients is that it:

a. helps them understand what nurses do.

b. increases collaborative practice and job satisfaction.

c. ensures efficient use of nursing time and resources.

d. helps ensure quality care that meets individual needs.

a
Knowledge
Safety: Management
of Care

17-15 The nursing process benefits individual nurses primarily by:

a. improving job satisfaction.

b. helping them to meet unique client needs.

c. making staffing assignments easier.

d. conserving health care resources.

a
Comprehension
Assessment
Promotion:
Prevention and Early
Detection of Disease

17-16 In the assessing phase, the nurse collects data in order to:

a. identify nursing diagnoses.

b. confirm the medical diagnosis.

c. establish rapport with the client.

d. determine client responses to nursing interventions.

b
Comprehension
Assessment
Promotion:
Prevention and Early
Detection of Disease

17-17 An example of objective data is:

a. nausea.

b. vomiting.

c. joint pain.

d. headache.

c
Comprehension
Assessment
Promotion:
Prevention and Early
Detection of Disease

17-18 An example of subjective data is:

a. temperature of 101° F.

b. vomiting.

c. nausea.

d. BP 128/78.

d
Knowledge
Assessment
Promotion:
Prevention and Early
Detection of Disease

17-19 The primary source of data collection is the:

a. chart.

b. doctor.

c. family.

d. client.

b
Knowledge
Assessment
Promotion:
Prevention and Early
Detection of Disease

17-20 Observation includes noticing stimuli and:

a. interviewing the client to validate the data.

b. selecting, organizing, and interpreting the data.

c. developing a nursing diagnosis from the data.

d. measuring them against norms or standards.

c
Application
Assessment
Promotion:
Prevention and Early
Detection of Disease

17-21 Which of the following is an example of a nursing action in the assessing step of the nursing process?

a. The nurse observes that the client's pain was relieved by the medication administered.

b. The nurse changes the bed linens after the client spills milk in the bed.

c. The nurse asks the client how much lunch he ate.

d. The nurse works with the client to set goals and desired outcomes.

a
Application
Assessment
Promotion:
Prevention and Early
Detection of Disease

17-22 The client states, "My lips feel numb and I can't see very well." What is the type and source of this data?

a. subjective data from a primary source

b. objective data from a primary source

c. subjective data from a secondary source

d. objective data from a secondary source

b
Application
Assessment
Physiological:
Reduction of Risk
Potential

17-23 You are straining the client's urine and measuring the output. Which of the following should be recorded as objective data?

a. The client complained of abdominal pain this morning.

b. There were no stones in the client's strained urine.

c. The client stated, "It felt like I passed a stone."

d. The client said she didn't see any stones in the urine.

a
Knowledge
Assessment
Promotion:
Prevention and Early
Detection of Disease

17-24 Which assessment method is performed by using the senses, primarily the sense of sight?

a. observation

b. interviewing

c. examination

d. palpating

d
Knowledge
Assessment
Promotion:
Prevention and Early
Detection of Disease

17-25 During the assessing component of the nursing process, the primary reason for interviewing a client is to:

a. establish rapport.

b. teach needed information.

c. provide emotional therapy.

d. collect data.

b
Knowledge
Assessment
Promotion:
Prevention and Early
Detection of Disease

17-26 The nondirective interview is best for:

a. obtaining specific information quickly.

b. building rapport with the client.

c. enabling the nurse to control the interview.

d. limiting discussion.

c
Application
Assessment
Physiological::
Physiological
Adaptation

17-27 A client is admitted to the unit and assigned to you. The client is slightly pale; cool and sweating; and seems a little anxious. As the nurse you should:

a. help the client get settled, orient him to the room, wait until he is rested, and do the interview in the morning.

b. do the interview immediately, but direct the questions to the client's wife.

c. do the interview as soon as you can plan 15 to 20 minutes of uninterrupted time, intervening to relieve the client's anxiety at that time.

d. ask the charge nurse to interview the client since she is probably more experienced in handling anxiety than you are.

a
Application
Assessment
Promotion:
Prevention and Early
Detection of Disease

17-28 Which of the following statements or questions would be most likely to quickly elicit specific information?

a. "Where does it hurt?"

b. "Describe what you are feeling."

c. "How are you today?"

d. "What would you like to talk about?"

d
Application
Assessment
Promotion:
Prevention and Early
Detection of Disease

17-29 During an interview, the nurse asks the client, "Would you describe the support you can expect from your family?" The nurse should expect an answer that:

a. furnishes information to answer a specific question.

b. does not provide much information.

c. is one or two words long.

d. expresses feelings or provides details.

b
Application
Assessment
Promotion:
Prevention and Early
Detection of Disease

17-30 Which of the following is an example of a leading question?

a. "What has your doctor told you about your illness?"

b. "You are really excited about the baby, aren't you?"

c. "How long have you had this symptom?"

d. "How do you feel about that?"

c
Application
Assessment
Promotion:
Prevention and Early
Detection of Disease

17-31 Most people feel comfortable when they are three to four feet from their interviewer. Knowing this, how should the nurse individualize the interview for an Asian male client?

a. The nurse should begin by sitting four feet from the bed in a position that allows for direct eye contact.

b. The nurse should begin by standing a little closer than usual, perhaps two feet from the bed.

c. The nurse should begin by sitting at least four feet from the bed and avoiding direct eye contact.

d. The nurse should begin by standing at the foot of the bed.

a
Application
Assessment
Psychosocial:
Psychosocial
Adaptation

17-32 The nurse asks a client, "Did your husband hit you?" This is an example of a(n):

a. closed question.

b. open-ended question.

c. leading question.

d. neutral question.

a
Application
Assessment
Promotion:
Prevention and Early
Detection of Disease

17-33 During which part of the interview would it be best to ask, "Who won the ball game last night?"

a. opening

b. body

c. closing

d. orientation

b
Application
Assessment
Promotion:
Prevention and Early
Detection of Disease

17-34 During which part of the interview should the nurse ask the client questions about her current illness?

a. opening

b. body

c. closing

d. rapport-building

d
Comprehension
Assessment
Promotion:
Prevention and Early
Detection of Disease

17-35 The nurse first assesses the client's overall appearance, then respiratory status, circulation, skin condition, nervous system, and so on. Which physical assessment approach is this nurse using?

a. head-to-toe
b. anthropometric
c. screening
d. body systems

b
Comprehension
Assessment
Safety: Management
of Care

17-36 The advantage of using a nursing conceptual model to organize data collection is that nursing frameworks:

a. focus on abnormalities of body systems.
b. provide for collecting patterns of functional and dysfunctional behaviors.
c. focus mainly on developmental concerns.
d. cluster data according to a hierarchy of client needs.

c
Application
Assessment
Promotion:
Prevention and Early
Detection of Disease

17-37 Which of the following data should be validated?

a. The client tells you he is 36 years old.
b. The chart indicates that the client weighs 145 pounds.
c. The client says, "I feel like I have a fever."
d. You count the client's pulse at 84. It was 80 yesterday.

c
Comprehension
Assessment
Promotion:
Prevention and Early
Detection of Disease

17-38 During which part of the interview would the nurse be most likely to say to the client, "Do you have any more questions concerning your hospital stay?"

a. opening
b. body
c. closing
d. orientation

a
Comprehension
Assessment
Promotion:
Prevention and Early
Detection of Disease

17-39 Nursing assessment is done in order to:

a. identify health problems and plan client care.
b. offer suggestions to the client for improving coping skills.
c. determine the cause of the client's disease.
d. demonstrate nursing autonomy.

d
Application
Assessment
Promotion:
Prevention and Early
Detection of Disease

17-40 Which of the following is an example of subjective data?

a. You see that the client's face is red.
b. You palpate a hard abdomen.
c. The nursing assistant tells you that the client was incontinent of urine.
d. The client says he feels nauseated.

c
Comprehension
Analysis/Diagnosis
Physiological:
Physiological
Adaptation

18-1 A nursing diagnosis focuses on:

a. the pathophysiology of the client's illness.

b. describing the client's symptoms.

c. the client's responses to stress, disease, or injury.

d. describing the client's needs.

a
Comprehension
Analysis/Diagnosis
Physiological:
Physiological
Adaptation

18-2 Which of the following diagnoses is stated as a potential health problem?

a. Risk for Injury

b. Anxiety

c. Sleep Pattern Disturbance

d. Ineffective Individual Coping

b
Comprehension
Analysis/Diagnosis
Physiological:
Physiological
Adaptation

18-3 A client has a fractured hip. 'Fractured hip' is a:

a. nursing diagnosis.

b. medical diagnosis.

c. collaborative diagnosis.

d. potential problem.

b
Application
Analysis/Diagnosis
Promotion:
Prevention and Early
Detection of Disease

18-4 Which of the following bests applies to the description "normal fragile, intact skin of a newborn infant?" It poses a(n):

a. actual health problem.

b. wellness diagnosis.

c. collaborative health problem.

d. possible nursing diagnosis.

d
Application
Analysis/Diagnosis
Promotion: Growth
and Development
Through the Life
Span

18-5 In evaluating a child's blood pressure reading, the nurse considers the child's age. This is an example of:

a. clustering data.

b. determining gaps in the data.

c. differentiating cues and inferences.

d. comparing data against standards.

c
Knowledge
Analysis/Diagnosis
Safety: Management
of Care

18-6 Formulating nursing diagnoses and client strengths is a joint function of the:

a. nurse and physician.

b. client and family.

c. nurse and client.

d. physician and client.

a
Knowledge
Analysis/Diagnosis
Safety: Management
of Care

18-7   A nursing diagnosis is a problem for which the nurse can:

a.   order definitive treatment or prevention interventions.

b.   order all necessary treatments and interventions.

c.   provide only dependent interventions.

d.   only monitor to detect onset of a physiological complication.

b
Comprehension
Analysis/Diagnosis
Safety: Management
of Care

18-8   A collaborative problem is one for which the independent nursing actions
are primarily used to:

a.   prevent and treat.

b.   prevent and detect.

c.   diagnose and treat.

d.   teach and counsel.

b
Comprehension
Analysis/Diagnosis
Physiological:
Physiological
Adaptation

18-9   "The client will probably develop pneumonia if certain independent
nursing actions are not carried out." This constitutes a(n) _____
nursing diagnosis.

a.   actual

b.   risk

c.   possible

d.   wellness

a
Knowledge
Analysis/Diagnosis
Physiological:
Physiological
Adaptation

18-10   Identify the italicized part of this nursing diagnosis: *Impaired Skin
Integrity: Excoriation* related to prolonged exposure to ammonia
secondary to incontinence of urine.

a.   problem

b.   cue

c.   etiology

d.   contributing factor

c
Knowledge
Analysis/Diagnosis
Physiological:
Physiological
Adaptation

18-11   Identify the italicized part of this nursing diagnosis: Impaired Skin
Integrity: Excoriation related to *prolonged exposure to ammonia secondary to
incontinence of urine.*

a.   cue

b.   problem

c.   etiology

d.   diagnostic label

d
Comprehension
Analysis/Diagnosis
Safety: Management
of Care

18-12   In the diagnostic process, the nurse should:

a.   use only objective data to infer problems.

b.   focus on identifying the disease process.

c.   be concerned only with actual problems.

d.   look for patterns and deviations from normal.

d
Comprehension
Analysis/Diagnosis
Safety: Management
of Care

18-13   If a nurse does not have enough data to confirm an actual nursing diagnosis of Anxiety, the nurse should write a:

a. risk nursing diagnosis.

b. collaborative problem.

c. wellness diagnosis.

d. possible nursing diagnosis.

d
Application
Analysis/Diagnosis
Safety: Safety and
Infection Control

18-14   For the nursing diagnosis Risk for Injury: Falls related to impaired vision, what is/are the risk factor(s)?

a. high risk

b. injury

c. falls

d. impaired vision

a
Comprehension
Analysis/Diagnosis
Safety: Management
of Care

18-15   It is important to identify the etiology of a nursing diagnosis because the etiology:

a. enables the nurse to individualize interventions for a particular client.

b. describes the pathophysiology of the client's disease.

c. determines whether the problem is actual or potential.

d. includes the defining characteristics of the diagnosis.

b
Application
Analysis/Diagnosis
Physiological:
Physiological
Adaptation

18-16   The nurse observes the individual cues of groaning, grimacing, and refusing to move and concludes that as a group, they represent the NANDA label of Pain. This type of reasoning is:

a. deductive.

b. inductive.

c. interpretive.

d. analytic.

a
Application
Analysis/Diagnosis
Psychosocial:
Coping and
Adaptation

18-17   A client withholds information out of anxiety and embarrassment. In this case, if the nurse makes a diagnostic error it would probably be because of:

a. incomplete data.

b. generalizing from experience.

c. identifying with the client.

d. lack of clinical experience.

b
Application
Analysis/Diagnosis
Physiological:
Physiological
Adaptation

18.18   Which of the following is an inference rather than a cue?

a. blood pressure is 160/100

b. rapid pulse

c. urine output = 400 cc

d. client states he is afraid of surgery

b
Application
Analysis/Diagnosis
Promotion: Growth
and Development
Through the Life
Span

18-19 The nurse is caring for a single mother who has just given birth to her second child. The nurse cannot imagine being responsible for raising a child alone and knows she would make sure to use a reliable birth control method. The nurse concludes that her client lacks knowledge of birth control methods. Which of the following actions will best help the nurse to avoid diagnostic error in this situation?

a. acquiring more clinical experience

b. verifying the hypothesis with the client

c. having a working knowledge of what is normal

d. consulting resources (for example, nursing journals)

c
Application
Analysis/Diagnosis
Safety: Management
of Care

18-20 Which of the following is stated in the format of a collaborative problem?

a. Risk for Pneumonia related to immobility and pain

b. Complication of Surgery: Pneumonia

c. Potential Complication of Surgery: Pneumonia

d. Pneumonia related to immobility and pain secondary to surgery

c
Comprehension
Analysis/Diagnosis
Safety: Management
of Care

18-21 Of the four components of a NANDA diagnostic label, which one is the most similar to a client's 'signs and symptoms'?

a. title (or label)

b. definition

c. defining characteristics

d. label definition

d
Application
Analysis/Diagnosis
Physiological:
Physiological
Adaptation

18-22 Which of the following diagnostic statements uses the PES format?

a. Risk for Impaired Skin Integrity as manifested by poor skin turgor and immobility

b. Risk for Impaired Skin Integrity related to decreased peripheral circulation secondary to diabetes

c. Altered Nutrition: Less than Body Requirements related to anorexia and dyspnea

d. Altered Nutrition: More than Body Requirements related to eating when depressed as manifested by weight of 50% more than recommended for height and client report of food intake of more than 3000 calories per day

18-23   What is wrong with the diagnostic statement Risk for Fluid Volume Deficit related to loss of fluid during surgery and possible post-op hemorrhage?

a. The nurse cannot prescribe the interventions necessary for goal achievement.

b. The nurse cannot prescribe the interventions for monitoring and detection.

c. It has more than one etiology.

d. It is stated in legally questionable terms.

18-24   Which of the following is an accepted variation in format for a nursing diagnosis?

a. including more than one problem

b. writing 'unknown etiology' when the cause is unknown

c. writing a diagnosis in which the two parts mean the same thing

d. using a medical diagnosis as the etiology

18-25   Which of the following descriptors could be used in stating the problem part of a nursing diagnosis?

a. Crying

b. Possible Anxiety

c. temperature 101° F

d. intake 750 cc in 8 hours

19 PLANNING

c
Comprehension
Planning
Safety: Management
of Care

19-1 Which of the following activities is a part of the planning phase of the nursing process?

a. formulating a nursing diagnosis

b. analyzing client data

c. developing client goals/desired outcomes

d. carrying out a nursing order

a
Knowledge
Planning
Safety: Management
of Care

19-2 Discharge planning should begin:

a. upon admission.

b. the day before discharge.

c. 24 hours after admission.

d. when the client is well.

b
Knowledge
Planning
Safety: Management
of Care

19-3 The client returns from surgery, and the nurse writes a nursing order on his care plan for "turning every 2 hours." A nursing order is a(n):

a. interpretation of a medical order.

b. independent nursing action.

c. component of a collaborative desired outcome.

d. standard of care.

d
Application
Planning
Physiological: Basic
Care and Comfort

19-4 What is missing from the following desired outcome? "Will ambulate with a walker by 6/1."

a. client behavior

b. target time

c. conditions or modifiers

d. performance criterion

a
Application
Planning
Physiological: Basic
Care and Comfort

19-5 What is wrong with the following nursing order? "10/31. Encourage ambulation ad lib. J. Jones, RN."

a. not specific enough

b. it is a dependent action

c. too wordy

d. unrealistic

b
Application
Planning
Physiological: Basic
Care and Comfort

19-6   What is wrong with the following desired outcome? "Client will be able to climb one flight of stairs without shortness of breath."

a. Nothing is wrong.

b. No target time is given.

c. It is not measurable.

d. Behavioral terms are not used.

d
Application
Planning
Physiological: Basic
Care and Comfort

19-7   "Client will establish normal bowel elimination patterns within 2 months." This is an example of a:

a. nursing diagnosis.

b. nursing order.

c. short-term goal.

d. long-term goal.

b
Application
Planning
Promotion:
Prevention and Early
Detection of Disease

19-8   Which of the following is a correctly written and measurable desired outcome?

a. The client will be adequately hydrated by May 6.

b. The client will lose 5 pounds within the next 2 weeks.

c. The nurse will provide emotional support at least 3 times each day.

d. The client will walk better after resting for 10 minutes.

a
Application
Planning
Physiological: Basic
Care and Comfort

19-9   Which of these is a specific, measurable desired outcome?

a. Has daily bowel movement beginning on 10/21.

b. Understands diabetic diet by dismissal.

c. Regains optimum state of health by 10/21.

d. Achieves good post-op recovery by day 3.

b
Application
Planning
Physiological: Basic
Care and Comfort

19-10   The client's nursing diagnosis is Risk for Impaired Skin Integrity related to pressure and immobility secondary to pain and presence of cast. Which of the following desired outcomes must be included in the care plan?

a. Client will be able to turn himself by day 3.

b. Skin will remain intact and without redness during hospital stay.

c. Client will state pain relieved within 30 minutes after medication.

d. Pressure will be prevented by turning every 2 hours.

c
Comprehension
Planning
Safety: Management
of Care

19-11   Independent nursing orders on the care plan state the specific activities needed to:

a. carry out the medical regimen.

b. follow hospital policies.

c. help the client achieve his or her goals.

d. formulate a nursing diagnosis.

19-12 For a possible nursing diagnosis, the nursing interventions will be concerned mainly with:

a. client teaching.

b. maintaining the client's usual patterns.

c. collection of additional data.

d. preventing additional problems.

19-13 For a risk nursing diagnosis, the nursing interventions will be concerned mainly with:

a. relieving the symptoms.

b. client teaching for self-care.

c. carrying out the medical orders.

d. preventing and observing for symptoms.

19-14 The nurse should take the initiative in setting priorities when:

a. the client is indigent or uneducated.

b. a life-threatening situation occurs.

c. there is a conflict in client and nurse values.

d. the client is angry with the staff.

19-15 Goals can be derived from both the problem and etiology of a nursing diagnosis; however, at least one goal must be derived from the:

a. client problem.

b. etiology.

c. defining characteristics.

d. risk factors.

19-16 The broad goal for a client is to maintain a normal blood sugar level. Which of the following is a correctly written desired outcome?

a. The client will have adequate urinary output during the shift.

b. The client will have no alteration in skin integrity during hospitalization.

c. The client will have at each ac and hs check a blood glucose reading of 80–120.

d. The client will have no decrease in peripheral circulation by discharge.

d
Comprehension
Planning
Safety: Management
of Care

19-17 What is the primary disadvantage of using preprinted, standardized care plans, standards of care, and protocols?

a. Standards of care do not provide enough detail for the nurse.

b. Standardized care plans are too time-consuming to use on a busy unit.

c. Nurses who follow a standardized agency plan are not likely to achieve acceptable standards of care.

d. The nurse may overlook unique client needs that are not addressed by the plans.

d
Comprehension
Planning
Safety: Management
of Care

19-18 When consulting with other health care personnel regarding client-related issues, the nurse must:

a. provide the consultant with a detailed nursing history.

b. provide the consultant with the client's nursing care plan.

c. obtain permission from the client.

d. identify the specific problem.

b
Knowledge
Planning
Safety: Management
of Care

19-19 Which of the following is considered a multidisciplinary (collaborative) plan of care?

a. nursing care plan

b. critical pathway

c. standards of care

d. model (standard) care plan

c
Application
Planning
Psychosocial:
Coping and
Adaptation

19-20 What is missing from the following nursing order? "Monitor for verbalization of interest in group activities. S. Jiminez, RN."

a. action verb

b. rationale

c. time element

d. content area

d
Comprehension
Planning
Safety: Management
of Care

19-21 Nursing care plans should include all of the following *except* what?

a. preventative actions

b. orders for on-going assessment

c. discharge teaching needs

d. all the steps of a standard procedure

19-22   Which of the following is a goal?

    a.   The client will gain 2 lbs by day 3.

    b.   The client will identify four favorite foods.

    c.   The client will list five favorite beverages.

    d.   The client's nutritional status will improve.

19-23   According to the Nursing Outcomes Classification, an indicator is:

    a.   a goal.

    b.   a measure.

    c.   the desired outcome.

    d.   a taxonomy.

19-24   Desired outcomes are similar to:

    a.   goals.

    b.   indicators.

    c.   rationales.

    d.   criteria.

19-25   When writing goals, which of the following actions is *not* necessary for the nurse to do?

    a.   Make the goals client-specific.

    b.   Evaluate the goals in relation to the client's value system.

    c.   Make sure the desired outcomes are realistic for the client's abilities.

    d.   Identify nursing actions to meet the goals.

20-1 In the implementing step of the nursing process, the nurse:

    a. puts the care plan into action.

    b. determines whether desired outcomes have been achieved.

    c. assesses the health status of the client.

    d. identifies available nursing resources.

20-2 Which statement describes an independent nursing action?

    a. It is a nursing action carried out under the supervision of a physician.

    b. It is a nursing action performed jointly with another member of the health care team.

    c. It is a nursing action performed according to agency policies and procedures.

    d. It is a nursing action initiated as a result of the nurse's own knowledge and skills.

20-3 The first three steps of the nursing process (assessing, diagnosing, and planning) are the basis for the _____ nursing interventions performed during the implementing step.

    a. dependent

    b. independent

    c. collaborative

    d. preventive

20-4 Which of the following statements about nursing interventions is true?

    a. They are activities that the nurse initiates independently.

    b. They include all direct care that a nurse gives to a client.

    c. They include only those treatment activities ordered by a physician.

    d. They involve the care that is given as a result of nursing diagnoses.

20-5 While helping a client walk to the bathroom, the nurse observes that the client looks pale and is beginning to perspire heavily. She helps him back to bed, takes his vital signs, and records them on the graphic record at the bedside. Which activities constitute *reassessment*?

    a. helping the client walk to the bathroom

    b. recording the vital signs

    c. helping the client back to bed

    d. noting the pallor and taking the vital signs

c
Application
Implementation
Safety: Management
of Care

20-6 The nurse decides to allow the client's two-year-old granddaughter to visit before his open heart surgery. What type of implementation is this?

a. interpersonal
b. technical
c. cognitive
d. evaluative

b
Application
Implementation
Physiological:
Reduction of Risk
Potential

20-7 A client who had abdominal surgery yesterday is lying rigidly in bed and does not want to move. The nurse provides instruction on the importance of moving to prevent pneumonia. This is an example of:

a. critical thinking.
b. interpersonal skills.
c. performing tasks.
d. psychomotor skills.

c
Application
Implementation
Physiological: Basic
Care and Comfort

20-8 The nurse informs the radiology department that the client is too weak to travel by wheelchair and needs to be transported by stretcher. Which phase of the nursing process is this?

a. assessment
b. planning
c. implementation
d. evaluation

b
Knowledge
Implementation
Safety: Management
of Care

20-9 Which kind of assessment occurs along with implementation?

a. admission assessment
b. ongoing assessment
c. discharge assessment
d. medical assessment

a
Application
Implementation
Physiological: Basic
Care and Comfort

20-10 While feeding a client, the nurse observes the client grimacing and having difficulty swallowing. The nurse asks the client if his throat is still sore. The client nods his head and refuses to eat any more. The nurse takes the tray away and records the incident in the client's chart. Which of these actions clearly demonstrates implementing and *not* reassessing?

a. the nurse feeding the client
b. the client having difficulty swallowing
c. the nurse asking if the client's throat is still sore
d. the nurse observing that the client is grimacing

c
Application
Implementation
Safety: Safety and
Infection Control

20-11 A client tells his nurse he needs to use the bedside commode. He is very large and weak and usually requires the support of two nurses to make the transfer. The nurse calls for help, but no one is available. The client states, "I can't wait. If I don't get up right now, I'll go in the bed." What should the nurse do?

a. Encourage the client to wait, and continue to call for help.

b. Leave the client's room and go obtain clean bed linen.

c. Help the client onto a bedpan, if the nurse can safely do so alone.

d. Help the client up to the commode, advising him to let the nurse know sooner next time.

d
Application
Implementation
Physiological: Basic
Care and Comfort

20-12 When deciding the best time to ambulate a postoperative client, which implementation skill is the nurse using?

a. interpersonal

b. technical

c. psychomotor

d. cognitive

a
Application
Implementation
Physiological:
Reduction of Risk
Potential

20-13 A nurse is to administer an intramuscular injection to a very emaciated (thin) woman. The nurse decides to use a 1-inch needle instead of the usual 1.5-inch needle. Which implementing guideline does this illustrate?

a. Nursing actions should be adapted to the individual client.

b. Nursing actions should be holistic.

c. Nursing actions require teaching and support.

d. Nursing actions should respect the client's dignity.

b
Application
Implementation
Safety: Management
of Care

20-14 Which activity occurs in the implementing phase of the nursing process?

a. formulating a nursing diagnosis

b. recording nursing interventions

c. writing the nursing orders

d. comparing client responses to the desired outcomes

c
Knowledge
Implementation
Safety: Management
of Care

20-15 In the nursing process, which step comes after planning?

a. assessment

b. diagnosis

c. implementation

d. evaluation

d
Application
Implementation
Physiological:
Pharmacological and
Parenteral Therapies

20-16 A physician has written an order for morphine, 10 mg. The nurse believes the dosage is unsafe for the client because he is thin, elderly, and has shallow, slow respirations. The nurse should:

a. give the morphine and chart his reservations about it.
b. waste the morphine and chart that it was given.
c. give the morphine and chart it in the usual way.
d. call the physician and discuss the order and his reservations about it.

d
Knowledge
Evaluation
Safety: Management
of Care

20-17 The most important purpose of the evaluation step of the nursing process is to:

a. identify the client's strengths.
b. carry out the nursing orders.
c. identify effective nursing actions.
d. determine if client goals have been met.

a
Application
Evaluation
Physiological:
Pharmacological and
Parenteral Therapies

20-18 The nurse returns 30 minutes after administering an antiemetic to ask the client if her nausea has subsided. This is an example of _____ evaluation.

a. ongoing
b. intermittent
c. terminal
d. unnecessary

b
Comprehension
Evaluation
Safety: Management
of Care

20-19 Which of the following actions is part of the evaluation process?

a. planning nursing strategies
b. reexamining the client's care plan
c. identifying available resources
d. carrying out nursing orders

a
Knowledge
Evaluation
Safety: Management
of Care

20-20 The first component of the evaluation process actually occurs in the planning step of the nursing process. What is it?

a. identifying desired outcomes.
b. reviewing the client's care planning
c. relating nursing actions to client outcomes
d. comparing reassessment data with desired outcomes

d
Comprehension
Evaluation
Physiological:
Physiological
Adaptation

20-21 If the nurse determines that a client goal (desired outcome) has not been met, the next step is to:

a. notify the physician.
b. discontinue the care planning.
c. continue current nursing interventions until the goal is met.
d. reexamine the care plan to see if it needs to be revised.

d
Knowledge
Evaluation
Safety: Management
of Care

20-22　The term *quality assurance* implies that:

　　a.　clients receive optimum levels of care.

　　b.　records have been examined or reviewed.

　　c.　peer review of nursing care has been done.

　　d.　an effort has been made to evaluate and ensure quality health care.

c
Knowledge
Evaluation
Safety: Management
of Care

20-23　The term *peer review* describes a(n):

　　a.　evaluation of a client's record after discharge.

　　b.　examination of agency services.

　　c.　review of practices by an equal.

　　d.　retrospective audit.

b
Application
Evaluation
Physiological: Basic
Care and Comfort

20-24　The nurse makes the following entry in the client's record: "Goal not met; client refuses to breastfeed due to dry, cracked nipples." Since the goal has not been met, the nurse should:

　　a.　reassign the client to another nurse.

　　b.　reexamine the nursing orders.

　　c.　notify the physician.

　　d.　write a new nursing diagnosis.

b
Application
Evaluation
Safety: Management
of Care

20-25　During a client's hospitalization, the quality assurance nurse reviews the interventions that the nurses have documented on the chart. This is an example of a(n):

　　a.　terminal audit.

　　b.　concurrent audit.

　　c.　retrospective audit.

　　d.　outcome audit.

c
Application
Evaluation
Physiological:
Physiological
Adaptation

20-26　A desired outcome on a client's care plan reads, "Client will state three signs of hypoglycemia by discharge." When the nurse evaluates the client's progress, the client is able to state that weakness and perspiration are signs of hypoglycemia. Which statement would be an appropriate evaluation statement?

　　a.　Client understands the signs of hypoglycemia.

　　b.　Goal met; client cited weakness and perspiration as signs of hypoglycemia.

　　c.　Goal not met; client able to name only two signs of hypoglycemia.

　　d.　Goal not met.

d
Application
Implementation
Safety: Management
of Care

20-27 Which nursing action would be appropriate to delegate to an unlicensed nursing assistant?

a. giving regularly scheduled intravenous medications

b. analyzing the lab results of a client with pneumonia

c. evaluating the desired outcomes for a postoperative client

d. taking the temperature of all the clients on one side of the hall

b
Application
Evaluation
Safety: Management
of Care

20-28 During the second week of February, all clients admitted to the preoperative unit were asked if it would be helpful to have a clock and calendar in the room. This is a type of:

a. retrospective audit.

b. structure evaluation.

c. process evaluation.

d. outcome evaluation.

21 DOCUMENTING AND REPORTING

b
Comprehension
Assessment
Safety: Management
of Care

21-1 A client was admitted to your unit following an automobile accident. If you are using a source-oriented medical record, where would you find his date of birth recorded?

    a. nurses' notes

    b. admission sheet

    c. social service record

    d. physician's order sheet

d
Comprehension
Assessment
Safety: Management
of Care

21-2 In a source-oriented medical record, where should the nurse look to find out the amount of a client's previous 24-hour urine output?

    a. physician's progress notes

    b. nurses' notes

    c. diagnostic reports

    d. special flowsheets

b
Comprehension
Implementation
Safety: Management
of Care

21-3 The client has been in the hospital for two days. After taking her vital signs, where in the permanent record would you chart this data?

    a. nurses' notes

    b. graphic sheet

    c. bedside worksheet

    d. admission sheet

c
Knowledge
Implementation
Safety: Management
of Care

21-4 Information in a client's chart may be considered inadmissible as court evidence when:

    a. the writing is not legible.

    b. there are missing pages.

    c. the client objects to its use.

    d. the client's physician refuses permission.

a
Knowledge
Planning
Safety: Management
of Care

21-5 Which of the following is a benefit of the automated client care planning system?

    a. Current information concerning the client can be updated easily.

    b. The computer can arrive at a nursing diagnosis from assessment data.

    c. The number of nurses required to give nursing care can be reduced.

    d. The cost of hospitalization for the client is reduced.

d
Application
Implementation
Safety: Management
of Care

21-6   Your client insists she is leaving the hospital, even although her doctor has said she cannot go. She refuses to sign the AMA form to release the hospital from responsibility for her actions. What should the nurse do?

a.   Call security and have them persuade her to sign.

b.   Treat this as a normal discharge, but do not accompany her to the exit.

c.   Explain to her that she will need to wait until you can call the nursing supervisor.

d.   Document on the form that she will not sign and have it witnessed by another health professional.

c
Knowledge
Evaluation
Safety: Management
of Care

21-7   What is the major disadvantage of narrative charting (compared to other types of charting)?

a.   Too many abbreviations are used.

b.   Information is recorded in chronological order.

c.   Information related to a specific problem is found in multiple places.

d.   The nurse spends more time charting and less time on client care.

d
Comprehension
Implementation
Safety: Management
of Care

21-8   Which of the following statements best describes focus charting?

a.   It limits information to physiological problems.

b.   It eliminates repetitive charting of routine care by charting only exceptions to norms.

c.   It minimizes the use of flowsheets.

d.   It organizes progress notes by data, action, and response.

b
Comprehension
Implementation
Safety: Management
of Care

21-9   A documentation system in which only significant findings or deviations from norms are recorded is called:

a.   narrative charting.

b.   charting by exception.

c.   SOAP charting.

d.   focus charting.

c
Knowledge
Evaluation
Safety: Management
of Care

21-10   The purpose of a nursing audit is to:

a.   provide data for research.

b.   disseminate information to health care providers.

c.   compare actual nursing care to established standards.

d.   study a client's illness and treatment regimen closely.

a
Application
Assessment
Safety: Management
of Care

21-11 In which category of SOAP charting would the nurse look to find out whether a client had complained of nausea?

a. subjective data

b. objective data

c. assessment

d. plan

a
Application
Assessment
Safety: Management
of Care

21-12 An RN returns to work following a vacation and is assigned to new clients. Where can the RN quickly find accurate, up-to-date information on each client?

a. Kardex

b. previous nurse's worksheet

c. admission sheet of each client

d. computer printout of hospital census

d
Application
Implementation
Safety: Management
of Care

21-13 Which of the following types of information would be most informative and should be given in the change-of-shift report?

a. Vital signs are BP 120/80, pulse 72, and respirations 16.

b. Client is alert and in good spirits.

c. Chest x-ray taken 2 days ago was negative.

d. Client voided 400 cc of yellow urine 4 hours after the urinary catheter was removed.

d
Knowledge
Implementation
Safety: Management
of Care

21-14 After charting your nurses' notes after those of the previous shift, you discover you have made an error. How should you correct it?

a. Blot or use whiteout on the incorrect entry.

b. Recopy that page of nurses' notes.

c. Erase the error and fill in the correct information.

d. Draw a line through the error and write 'Error' and your initials above it.

d
Application
Implementation
Safety: Management
of Care

21-15 A client on your unit is deteriorating but remains alert and oriented. Three days after admission, you notice that he seems depressed. He tells you, "I'm tired of being sick. I wish I could end it all." What is the most accurate and informative way to record this data in the nurses' notes?

a. Appears to be depressed, possibly suicidal.

b. Complains he is tired of being ill and wants to die.

c. Does not want to live any longer because he is tired of being ill.

d. Client states, "I'm tired of being sick. I wish I could end it all."

21-16   A physician writes the abbreviated order DAT. What does it mean?

a.   discharge assessment today

b.   don't ambulate today

c.   diet as tolerated

d.   daily activities as tolerated

21-17   In which component of the problem-oriented medical record would the nurse find the medical or nursing orders?

a.   database

b.   problem list

c.   plan of care

d.   progress notes

21-18   Which of the following is a charting error?

a.   using a black ballpoint pen

b.   hand printing your nurses' notes because your cursive writing is hard to read

c.   signing the nurses' note that the relief nurse wrote about her client while she was at lunch

d.   including the date and time in each of chart entry

21-19   When health care records are reviewed to find out the annual number of births, the records are fulfilling the purpose of:

a.   legal documentation.

b.   education.

c.   statistics.

d.   audit.

21-20   Which one of the following methods of conferring encourages client participation?

a.   change-of-shift report

b.   nursing care conference

c.   staff meeting

d.   nursing care rounds

21-21   The nurse charts, "NG tube irrigated with 25 cc normal saline." In the focus charting method, this entry goes under the:

a.   data.

b.   action.

c.   response.

d   plan.

b
Application
Implementation
Safety: Management
of Care

21-22 The physician has called with a telephone order for one of her clients. What should the RN do?

a. Write the order in the chart, and have the head nurse co-sign it.

b. Repeat the order back to the physician, then copy it onto the order sheet, indicating 'TO' for telephone order.

c. Explain to the physician that he cannot take the order but that he will page the nursing supervisor.

d. Copy the order onto the physician's order sheet, and sign the physician's name, copying her handwriting as closely as possible.

b
Application
Implementation
Physiological:
Pharmacological and
Parenteral Therapies

21-23 The order says to give the medication 'tid'. Which of the following schedules meets the ordered interval?

a. 9 A.M. and 9 P.M.

b. 9 A.M., 5 P.M., and 1 A.M.

c. 9 A.M., 3 P.M., 9 P.M., and 3 A.M.

d. 9 A.M. every other day

a
Comprehension
Evaluation
Safety: Management
of Care

21- 24 Which of the following is true regarding computerized documentation?

a. It enables data from multiple sources to be linked.

b. It increases the ability to maintain the confidentiality of the record.

c. It is easier to learn than traditional flowsheet and other chart forms.

d. Errors can be made more easily.

a
Knowledge
Planning
Safety: Management
of Care

21-25 Which care plan is used by health professionals from different disciplines and provides desired outcomes for clients with specific diagnoses?

a. critical pathway

b. Kardex

c. standardized care plan

d. problem-oriented record

a
Comprehension
Promotion: Growth
and Development
Through the Life
Span

22-1   In addition to occurring cephalocaudally, growth and development also:

     a.   has certain stages that are more critical than others.

     b.   begins as highly differentiated, or specific, and proceeds to more general responses.

     c.   proceeds from complex to simple acts, or from integrated to single acts.

     d.   occurs in different patterns for different people.

d
Comprehension
Analysis/Diagnosis
Promotion: Growth
and Development
Through the Life
Span

22-2   While observing neonates in the newborn nursery, you notice that their heads are disproportionately larger than their extremities. This illustrates the principle of:

     a.   differentiated development.

     b.   synchronous development.

     c.   proximal-to-distal growth and development.

     d.   cephalocaudal growth.

b
Knowledge
Assessment
Promotion: Growth
and Development
Through the Life
Span

22-3   *Development* may be defined as:

     a.   physical change with increase in size.

     b.   an increase in the complexity of function and skill progression.

     c.   a sequence of physical changes related to genetic influence.

     d.   the ability to handle environmental demands.

d
Knowledge
Assessment
Promotion: Growth
and Development
Through the Life
Span

22-4   Havighurst describes growth and development as occurring during six stages, each characterized by:

     a.   inner drives.

     b.   maturational readiness.

     c.   somatotypes.

     d.   developmental tasks.

b
Knowledge
Assessment
Promotion: Growth
and Development
Through the Life
Span

22-5   According to Havighurst, achieving emotional independence from parents and other adults is a developmental task of:

     a.   middle childhood.

     b.   adolescence.

     c.   early adulthood.

     d.   middle age.

b
Knowledge
Promotion: Growth
and Development
Through the Life
Span

22-6 Concepts of the unconscious mind, defense mechanisms, the id, and the ego were introduced by:

a. Sullivan.

b. Freud.

c. Piaget.

d. Erikson.

c
Application
Analysis/Diagnosis
Promotion: Growth
and Development
Through the Life
Span

22-7 A nurse agreed to present an inservice education program; however, instead of preparing her presentation , she went to a rap concert with several of her friends and had to reschedule the inservice program. Her behavior appears to have been governed by her:

a. libidinal instincts.

b. ego.

c. id.

d. superego.

a
Application
Analysis/Diagnosis
Promotion: Growth
and Development
Through the Life
Span

22-8 A nurse had to cancel a scheduled inservice education program because she went to a rap concert instead of preparing for the presentation . Later, she told her supervisor that she felt "really bad about not being prepared to do the inservice" and admitted that her priorities "got turned around." The apology was most likely governed by her:

a. superego.

b. ego.

c. id.

d. libido.

c
Knowledge
Assessment
Promotion: Growth
and Development
Through the Life
Span

22-9 According to Freud's psychoanalytic theory, the Electra complex refers to:

a. a male child's attraction to the mother and hostility toward the father

b. unresolved conflicts related to fixation in a stage

c. a female child's attraction to the father and hostility toward the mother

d. specific behaviors such as temper tantrums, nail biting, smoking, and alcoholism

c
Comprehension
Promotion: Growth
and Development
Through the Life
Span

22-10 In Freud's psychoanalytic theory, adaptive mechanisms result from conflicts between:

a. the id and the ego.

b. the conscience and the superego.

c. inner impulses.

d. libidinal instincts and social forces.

22-11 According to Freudian theory, the person who is probably fixated in the phallic stage of development is a(n):

a. obstinate man who loses his temper frequently and curses loudly.

b. man who has been fired from several jobs because he won't "take orders" from his supervisors.

c. alcoholic who also smokes heavily.

d. woman who has no close friends because she believes that there is no one she can trust.

22-12 A nurse using Erikson's framework could enhance the development of a 4-year-old client by:

a. being sure to keep all promises she makes to the child.

b. setting aside time to sit and talk with the child and encouraging him to express himself.

c. giving him small, achievable tasks that will build his self-confidence.

d. giving him tasks that must be carried out over a period of weeks, in order to promote perseverance.

22-13 Which theorist conceptualizes life as a series of crises, or as a sequence of levels of achievement, each of which must be completed successfully before moving on to the next stage?

a. Freud

b. Erikson

c. Gould

d. Kohlberg

22-14 According to Erikson, increased autonomy is a central issue in which of the following age groups?

a. early childhood (18 months to 3 years)

b. preschool (3 to 6 years)

c. adolescence (12 to 20 years)

d. young adulthood (20 to 40 years)

22-15 Which theorist expands most on the developmental tasks of old age?

a. Freud

b. Erikson

c. Gould

d. Peck

22-16 Which theory would be most useful in helping the nurse understand how children of various ages think, reason, and process information?

a. Erikson

b. Fowler

c. Gould

d. Piaget

22-17 Kohlberg's theory of moral development focuses on:

a. one's conscience and feelings such as guilt.

b. the reasons one gives for one's actions.

c. the morality of the decision (or action) itself.

d. virtues and character traits.

22-18 According to Fowler, the force that gives meaning to a person's life is:

a. love.

b. hope.

c. conscience.

d. faith.

22-19 A single developmental theory can be used in nursing to:

a. explain individual differences.

b. explain the growth and development of the whole human being.

c. provide psychosocial, sexual, and cognitive evaluation.

d. guide assessment and planning of nursing interventions.

22-20 Which of the following nursing interventions is most appropriate for 16-year-old's stage of growth and development?

a. controlling the client's environment so that her physical and psychological needs are met

b. accepting the client's chosen lifestyle, regardless of how risky it may seem to the nurse

c. helping the client to develop strategies for resolving conflicts with family and peers

d. helping the client's parents identify and meet any of the client's unmet needs

22-21 Using Freud's developmental theory as a framework, which of the following clients would suffer the most developmental impact?

a. a three-day-old boy having a circumcision

b. a two-year-old girl having a cleft palate repaired

c. a two-year-old girl having eye surgery

d. a four-year-old boy having a testicle repaired

b
Application
Planning
Promotion: Growth
and Development
Through the Life
Span

22-22   Which diversional activity would be best suited to a nine-year-old boy confined to bed in traction for broken legs?

a.   completing a small jigsaw puzzle of 12 pieces

b.   competing with himself in a handheld electronic game

c.   watching a game show on TV

d.   reading an adventure novel

b
Application
Assessment
Promotion: Growth
and Development
Through the Life
Span

22-23   Which of the following client statements made to the nurse best illustrates Kohlberg's stage of interpersonal concordance?

a.   "I report all my income so that I won't be audited ."

b.   "I will adhere to the exercise program so that I will please you."

c.   "I'm not using my cell phone in the hospital because of the safety policy."

d.   "I will comply with my doctor's orders if you will bring me a newspaper."

c
Application
Implementation
Promotion: Growth
and Development
Through the Life
Span

22-24   A three-year-old who is to be discharged tomorrow morning asks, "When can I go home?" A nurse who bases her response on the preconceptual phase of Piaget's cognitive development model would say:

a.   "You will go home when the doctor says you may."

b.   "You can go home tomorrow."

c.   "After you sleep tonight and wake up, you will go home."

d.   "You can go after your morning breathing treatment."

d
Application
Assessment
Promotion: Growth
and Development
Through the Life
Span

22-25   The nurse recognizes that a 65-year-old retired client has probably achieved Peck's status of ego differentiation when he says:

a.   "I'm very proud of my garden, but it's not like landing a big insurance account."

b.   "Selling insurance is a lifestyle; gardening is a hobby."

c.   "I wish that growing beautiful tomatoes was a good as selling a good insurance policy."

d.   "I was a good insurance salesman, but I am a great gardener."

23 DEVELOPMENT FROM CONCEPTION THROUGH ADOLESCENCE

d
Application
Analysis
Promotion: Growth
and Development
Through the Life
Span

23-1 Which of the following clients should the nurse recognize as having delayed development?

a. a six-week-old client with a posterior fontanel that is completely closed

b. a six-month-old client who can sit alone but cannot pull himself to a standing position

c. an eight-month-old client who stops an activity and looks at the parent when told "No!"

d. a 13- -month-old client who has not yet attempted to walk

b
Knowledge
Assessment
Promotion: Growth
and Development
Through the Life
Span

23-2 At the age of 6 months, an infant weighing 8.5 pounds at birth would be expected to weigh:

a. 12 to 13 pounds.

b. 17 to 18 pounds.

c. 19 to 20 pounds.

d. 21 to 22 pounds.

a
Application
Analysis
Promotion: Growth
and Development
Through the Life
Span

23-3 The nurse palpates the anterior fontanel of a 12-month-old client and finds that it is 1 cm. in diameter. The nurse should:

a. recognize this as a normal finding.

b. report this finding to the physician.

c. check the fontanel again the next day.

d. watch for signs of intracranial pressure.

b
Comprehension
Analysis
Promotion: Growth
and Development
Through the Life
Span

23-4 For an eight-month-old infant, which of the following behaviors should the nurse recognize as a possible problem that should be assessed more fully?

a. The infant is afraid of strangers.

b. The infant cannot sit without support.

c. The infant cries when scolded.

d. The infant cannot walk while holding onto furniture.

b
Knowledge
Promotion: Growth
and Development
Through the Life
Span

23-5 According to Erikson's theory of psychosocial development, the central task in infancy is the establishment of:

a. autonomy.

b. trust.

c. independence.

d. cognitive awareness.

b Application Planning Promotion: Growth and Development Through the Life Span	23-6	Which of the following would be an age-appropriate activity for a seven-month-old client hospitalized for treatment of a respiratory infection? a. watching an all-cartoon channel on TV b. playing with a soft rubber duck c. completing a simple puzzle d. playing with building blocks
a Application Assessment Promotion: Growth and Development Through the Life Span	23-7	At the age of 12 months, a child weighing 6.5 pounds at birth would be expected to weigh : a. 18 to 20 pounds b. 21 to 23 pounds. c. 25 to 27 pounds. d. 35 to 37 pounds.
d Comprehension Planning Promotion: Growth and Development Through the Life Span	23-8	To support adequate nutrition for a hospitalized toddler, the nurse should: a. insist the child eat some of each food on the plate. b. provide large servings so that food is left on plate when the child is done eating. c. let the child watch television or read to her while she eats. d. consult with the parents to determine the child's specific eating habits.
b Comprehension Analysis Psychosocial: Coping and Adaptation	23-9	A three-year-old was doing well with his toilet training until last week when his newborn sister came home from the hospital. Since then, he has started soiling his clothes and has become more demanding of his mother's attention. This behavior is most likely related to: a. a dislike for his new sibling. b. a regressive response to the stress of new family configuration. c. the imitation of the behaviors of his new sibling. d. being neglected by his mother, whose attention is on the new baby.
d Comprehension Assessment Promotion: Growth and Development Through the Life Span	23-10	Which of the following is typical behavior for a two-year-old child? a. sharing toys generously with other children b. engaging in cooperative play with peers c. patiently enduring frustrations or being told "no" d. imitating the words of others

c
Knowledge
Promotion: Growth
and Development
Through the Life
Span

23-11 The average age for completion of day and night bowel and bladder toilet training is:

a.   24 months.

b.   29 months.

c.   33 months.

d.   36 months.

d
Knowledge
Promotion: Growth
and Development
Through the Life
Span

23-12 According to Erikson, the central task of the preschooler (ages four to five years) is the development of:

a.   sexuality.

b.   morality.

c.   trust.

d.   initiative.

a
Knowledge
Promotion: Growth
and Development
Through the Life
Span

23-13 According to Freud, one of the adaptive mechanisms learned during the preschool years is:

a.   identification.

b.   sublimation.

c.   regression

d.   rationalization.

b
Knowledge
Assessment
Promotion: Growth
and Development
Through the Life
Span

23-14 According to Freudian theory, in the preschool child, feelings of love focus chiefly on:

a.   teachers.

b.   the opposite-sex parent.

c.   peers.

d.   the same-sex parent.

d
Knowledge
Assessment
Promotion: Growth
and Development
Through the Life
Span

23-15 During the phase of concrete operations (ages 7 to 11 years), which of the following behaviors would you expect a child to manifest?

a.   increase in egocentric interactions

b.   decrease in cooperative interactions

c.   development of magical thinking

d.   development of logical reasoning

a
Application
Analysis
Promotion: Growth
and Development
Through the Life
Span

23-16 Four school-age boys refuse to take part in a school yard prank. Which of them demonstrates Kohlberg's conventional level of moral development?

a. Boy # 1, who thinks, "My dad and mom would be so disappointed in me."

b. Boy # 2, who thinks, "We'll be sure to get caught if we do that. It's too risky."

c. Boy #3, who thinks, "We'll have to stay after school for a month, and my dad would yell at me for sure."

d. Boy # 4, who thinks, "If I stay out of this like the others, then maybe they'll like me more."

c
Knowledge
Assessment
Promotion: Growth
and Development
Through the Life
Span

23-17 Children learn to distinguish fantasy from fact during:

a. puberty.

b. preschool years.

c. school-age years.

d. adolescence.

c
Application
Assessment
Promotion: Growth
and Development
Through the Life
Span

23-18 When the nurse strokes the sole of a two-year old client's foot, the big toe rises and the other toes fan out. The nurse recognizes this as a:

a. Plantar reflex, which is abnormal for this age.

b. Stepping reflex, which is normal for this age.

c. Babinski reflex, which is abnormal for this age.

d. Moro reflex, with is normal for this age.

d
Comprehension
Analysis
Safety: Safety and
Infection Control

23-19 Which mother is following good safety practices for her six-month-old infant?

a. One who fastens the baby securely in a highchair before going outside to water the flowers.

b. One who puts the baby in bed and props the bottle so it is easily reached.

c. One who uses a crib with slats four inches apart.

d. One who uses a playpen with sides made of fine netting.

a
Comprehension
Assessment
Promotion: Growth
and Development
Through the Life
Span

23-20 The Apgar scoring system is used to assess the:

a. physical condition of the newborn.

b. cognitive development of children up to age 11.

c. psychosocial development of children up to adolescence.

d. musculoskeletal development of infants and toddlers.

d
Application
Evaluation
Psychosocial:
Coping and
Adaptation

23-21 For a nursing diagnosis of Altered Parenting related to parents' inability to meet infant's psychosocial needs, which behavior would best demonstrate the resolution of that problem?

a. The parents state that they now understand that infants need stimulation and can name some appropriate methods.

b. The parents can state the signs and symptoms of common infant illnesses.

c. The baby scores well on the Denver Developmental Screening Test.

d. The parents are meeting the infant's oral needs by giving him a pacifier when his sucking needs aren't completely met during feedings.

a
Comprehension
Planning
Promotion: Growth
and Development
Through the Life
Span

23-22 A 16-year-old with acne says, "I don't understand why I have it. I stopped eating chocolate, but it doesn't get any better." The nurse's reply should be based on the understanding that acne is typically a result of:

a. the sebaceous glands becoming active at puberty.

b. hormonal changes related to the menstrual cycle.

c. inadequate personal hygiene.

d. allergy to some environmental factor.

b
Knowledge
Promotion: Growth
and Development
Through the Life
Span

23-23 According to Erikson, the developmental task of adolescents is:

a. autonomy versus shame and doubt.

b. self-identity versus role confusion.

c. industry versus inferiority.

d. role acceptance versus role confusion.

c
Knowledge
Assessment
Promotion: Growth
and Development
Through the Life
Span

23-24 Which of the following is a secondary sexual characteristic?

a. ovulation

b. growth of the uterus

c. breast development

d. beginning of menstruation

Chapter 23 / Development from Conception Through Adolescence

d
Application
Implementation
Promotion: Growth
and Development
Through the Life
Span

23-25 A distraught parent has brought his 15-year-old son to the mental health center after finding him engaging in sexual activity with a male classmate. As the nurse, your most appropriate action is to:

a. refer the adolescent to a sex counselor who will help him to develop heterosexual behaviors.

b. explain to the parent that the sexual preference cannot be altered, and that he must try to accept the homosexuality.

c. ask to meet with the adolescent and his homosexual friend to assess the extent of their relationship.

d. reassure the parent that homosexual experimentation is common in adolescents, and it does not necessarily indicate a permanent sexual preference.

d
Application
Implementation
Promotion: Growth
and Development
Through the Life
Span

23-26 A 15-year-old girl does not want to go with her family on a trip they are planning, saying, "I'd rather stay here with my friends." The parents report that the adolescent spends free time with friends, and when at home, spends a lot of time in her room. Because the adolescent is often impatient and angry with them, the parents are perplexed when a math teacher tells them how charming and positive the adolescent is. The nurse should advise the parents to:

a. insist that the adolescent keep a detailed account of the time spent with the math teacher.

b. tell the adolescent that time with friends will be limited to an hour after school and for one day (or evening) on weekends, but no more.

c. make an appointment to have a counselor evaluate these behaviors, as they may be symptomatic of a personality disorder.

d. give consistent guidance, but ease up on restrictions and demands on her time, giving her as much freedom as she can handle.

c
Knowledge
Promotion: Growth
and Development
Through the Life
Span

23-27 Puberty is the:

a. process of establishing sexual identity.

b. acceptance of masculine or feminine sex roles.

c. stage in which sexual organs begin to grow and mature.

d. final stage of the growth and development process.

C
Application
Assessment
Promotion: Growth
and Development
Through the Life
Span

23-28 When a client's pregnancy ends in spontaneous abortion, the product of conception resembles a small baby, its red wrinkled skin covered with fine hair and vernix caseosa. The nurse assesses it to be a(n):

a. embryo, aged 8 weeks.

b. embryo, aged 12 weeks.

c. fetus, aged 4 months.

d. fetus, aged 8 months.

c
Application
Assessment
Promotion: Growth
and Development
Through the Life
Span

23-29   An infant is born with a heart rate of 92, its body pink, extremities blue, respirations regular, and crying while actively moving all extremities. Its Apgar score would be:

a.   4.

b.   6.

c.   8.

d.   10.

b
Application
Assessment
Physiological:
Physiological
Adaptation

23-30   A nine-month-old baby comes to the ER with seizures, an apical pulse of 76, and marked difficulty breathing. The physician notes retinal hemorrhages, but there are no external signs of injury. These are classic indications of:

a.   sudden infant death syndrome.

b.   shaken baby syndrome.

c.   failure to thrive.

d.   infant colic.

a
Application
Assessment
Promotion: Growth
and Development
Through the Life
Span

23-31   The school nurse notes that year-old female student has written the name of her 30-year-old history teacher all over her books and has surrounded the name with hearts. When the teenager describes her teacher as 'sexy' the nurse should be:

a.   amused by this normal crush on a teacher.

b.   troubled about the sexual attraction to an older man.

c.   alarmed as it indicates inappropriate sexual approaches by the teacher.

d.   alerted to probable sexual maladjustment in the teenager.

d
Application
Implementation
Promotion: Growth
and Development
Through the Life
Span

23-32   A teacher comes to the school nurse because she is worried that a 16-year-old female student seems depressed and may be suicidal. What is the most appropriate response by the nurse?

a.   "All teenagers are moody. This low period will pass."

b.   "You must bring her to the principal's office right away to be kept under observation."

c.   "I'll call the parents right away to come and get her."

d.   "I'll talk with her this afternoon and hear what she has to say."

c
Application
Implementation
Promotion: Growth
and Development
Through the Life
Span

23-33 Using Erikson as a framework, which activity would best support the developmental crisis of an eight-year-old boy hospitalized with asthma?

a. Allow him to choose his own foods from a menu to encourage autonomy.

b. Allow him to watch sports on TV to support identity.

c. Encourage him to build things out of Lego blocks to enhance industry.

d. Encourage him to color in a coloring book to stimulate initiative.

d
Comprehension
Promotion: Growth
and Development
Through the Life
Span

24-1   Which of the following is true about development in young adulthood?

a.   Effective communication and problem solving are essential when dealing with marital conflicts and adjustments, which are common in this period.

b.   Young adults generally accept their current life situation and are not likely to make significant changes during these years.

c.   Along with the stage of formal operations, the young adult becomes increasingly egocentric.

d.   Problem solving is difficult for young adults because of their cognitive stage and lack of life experience,.

b
Application
Assessment
Safety: Management
of Care

24-2   A 32-year-old single female is being discharged from the hospital in three days. She will have a full-length leg cast and will need assistance with transportation and shopping for the next six weeks. As the nurse planning her care, you would first:

a.   notify the person listed as next of kin and ask him or her to help the client establish a good support system.

b.   ask the client about her support system and significant others.

c.   refer the client to a vocational rehabilitation service to help her find a means of transportation.

d.   tell the client not to worry because several transportation services are available to her at little cost.

c
Knowledge
Safety: Safety and
Infection Control

24-3   Among young adults, the leading cause of death is:

a.   drowning.

b.   suicide.

c.   motor vehicle accidents.

d.   substance abuse.

d
Knowledge
Promotion: Growth
and Development
Through the Life
Span

24-4   Piaget believes that thinking in adulthood is characterized by:

a.   preoperational thought.

b.   intuitive thought.

c.   concrete operations.

d.   formal operations.

a
Comprehension
Assessment
Promotion:
Prevention and Early
Detection of Disease

24-5   The most important cancer screening test for young adult males is a(n):

    a.   monthly testicular self-examination.

    b.   monthly breast self-examination.

    c.   annual prostate examination.

    d.   annual chest x-ray.

c
Knowledge
Promotion:
Prevention and Early
Detection of Disease

24-6   Which health hazard is most likely to occur in young adulthood?

    a.   cancer

    b.   osteoporosis

    c.   hypertension

    d.   diabetes

b
Knowledge
Promotion: Growth
and Development
Through the Life
Span

24-7   According to Erikson, generativity versus stagnation is the developmental task of:

    a.   early adulthood.

    b.   middle adulthood.

    c.   early adolescence.

    d.   late adolescence.

b
Application
Analysis/Diagnosis
Promotion: Growth
and Development
Through the Life
Span

24-8   Which of the following adults is achieving one of the tasks of middle age according to Peck?

    a.   a 45-year-old divorced woman who has many friends, but will date only men who are handsome and sexually attractive

    b.   a 50-year-old woman who grieved when her son went away to college, but who is learning to play golf and is renewing her interest in her husband

    c.   a 55-year-old man who says, "Everything I need to know I learned in kindergarten. Don't talk to me about your radical ideas."

    d.   a 60-year-old widowed man who worries that he is not as strong and attractive as he was in his youth

a
Knowledge
Analysis/Diagnosis
Promotion: Growth
and Development
Through the Life
Span

24-9   Middle-aged adults are at risk for obesity because of a(n):

    a.   naturally occurring decrease in metabolism.

    b.   naturally occurring increase in appetite.

    c.   increase in estrogen (in women).

    d.   decrease in gastric juice secretions and free acid.

d
Comprehension
Assessment
Promotion: Growth
and Development
Through the Life
Span

24-10 Which of the following is characteristic of the health problems of older adults?

a. The proportion of acute conditions to chronic diseases increases.

b. Cardiac problems are the most common health problems.

c. Poverty ceases to contribute to their health problems because of Social Security and Medicare.

d. They are likely to be taking several prescribed medications, and the chance of adverse drug reactions increases.

d
Application
Analysis/Diagnosis
Promotion: Growth
and Development
Through the Life
Span

24-11 A 68-year-old woman frequently complains of being cold even although room temperature is 75 degrees. This is because many older people:

a. become confused and think it is much colder than it really is.

b. use this complaint to get attention .

c. have a malfunction of the heat-regulating mechanism in the brain.

d. have lost subcutaneous fat as they have aged.

c
Application
Implementation
Promotion: Growth
and Development
Through the Life
Span

24-12 A 70-year-old retired postal worker has developed brown spots on his hands and face, which his physician tells him are called lentigo senilus. The client asks, "Do you think these might be skin cancer? I haven't always had them." The nurse should answer:

a. "Don't be concerned. These are premalignant lesions and are easily cured."

b. "These are only premalignant lesions that have the potential of becoming cancerous."

c. "No, these are not cancer. Some people call them age spots. They are a normal change that occurs with aging."

d. "What did your doctor tell you about these lesions?"

c
Knowledge
Promotion: Growth
and Development
Through the Life
Span

24-13 A decrease in bone density along with an increased brittleness of the bones best describes:

a. osteoarthritis.

b. osteomalacia.

c. osteoporosis.

d. osteosarcoma.

b
Application
Implementation
Promotion: Growth
and Development
Through the Life
Span

24-14 When providing health teaching for an elderly client with osteoporosis, the nurse should:

a. encourage the client to prevent stress fractures by avoiding long walks.

b. instruct the client to eat foods high in calcium and vitamin D.

c. encourage the client to have a yearly bone scan.

d. instruct the client to take over-the-counter anti-inflammatory drugs for discomfort and joint stiffness.

c
Knowledge
Analysis/Diagnosis
Promotion: Growth
and Development
Through the Life
Span

24-15 Most elderly people have difficulty adjusting to near and far vision. This is because of eye changes that include:

a. diplopia.

b. bilateral deposition of orbital fat.

c. a relative inflexibility of the lens (presbyopia).

d. an increase in pupil diameter.

d
Comprehension
Implementation
Promotion: Growth
and Development
Through the Life
Span

24-16 Which intervention would be most helpful to an elderly person with impaired hearing?

a. Shout if the client does not seem to understand you.

b. Position yourself so that the client can read your lips.

c. Speak in a soft, high voice.

d. Use a low-pitched voice, saying each word distinctly.

c
Application
Assessment
Promotion: Growth
and Development
Through the Life
Span

24-17 In order to determine whether a client has accomplished Erikson's developmental task of integrity versus despair the nurse should assess the extent to which the client:

a. has achieved his lifelong goals and ambitions.

b. is making new friends to replace the expected loss of his loved ones.

c. feels comfortable and satisfied with the choices he has made in life.

d. is making changes in his personal appearance and manner of dress.

a
Comprehension
Promotion: Growth
and Development
Through the Life
Span

24-18 Disengagement theory explains psychosocial aging as:

a. a gradual decrease in interactions between the individual and society.

b. maintenance of preferred behaviors, habits, and values as one ages.

c. physical and mental activity to prevent the untoward effects of aging.

d. establishment of new activities to replace those no longer physically possible.

b
Application
Evaluation
Promotion: Growth
and Development
Through the Life
Span

24-19 A retired engineer who is adjusting satisfactorily to retirement should demonstrate which of the following behaviors?

a. He still sets the alarm clock and gets out of bed at 6:00 A.M., the same as when he was working.

b. He donates time as a volunteer at a local hospital and has renewed his interest in gardening.

c. He spends most of the day watching television and goes to bed by 8:30 P.M.

d. He stays in the kitchen with his wife while she cooks and follows her from room to room as she cleans the house, offering to help.

c
Comprehension
Promotion: Growth and Development Through the Life Span

24-20   Which of the following is characteristic of development in late adulthood?

  a. Intelligence declines.

  b. Most elderly people must relocate to nursing homes.

  c. Food and medical costs increase in proportion to total income.

  d. Women, as a group, receive more from pensions and government sources than men.

d
Knowledge
Analysis/Diagnosis
Promotion:
Prevention and Early Detection of Disease

24-21   The decline in health in middle age is primarily due to:

  a. normal processes of aging.

  b. acute illnesses.

  c. psychological depression.

  d. unhealthy lifestyles and habits.

a
Comprehension
Analysis/Diagnosis
Safety: Safety and Infection Control

24-22   When making a home visit to an elderly client, which of the following should the nurse recognize as a safety hazard that needs to be corrected?

  a. There is no light in the hallway between the bedroom and bathroom.

  b. When bathing, the client runs the cold water before the hot water.

  c. The client gets up slowly from the bed and stands briefly before walking.

  d. When walking to the store at night, the client states that he wears light-colored clothing.

b
Application
Assessment
Promotion:
Prevention and Early Detection of Disease

24-23   The home health nurse makes these four assessments on a 72-year-old female client. Which finding should be explored further, as it may be indicative of a developing problem?

  a. flat brown spots on the back of the client's hands

  b. a uterus that has increased in size and can be palpated

  c. inelastic skin

  d. occasional difficulty removing the tops from medicine bottles

a
Knowledge
Analysis/Diagnosis
Psychosocial:
Psychosocial
Adaptation

24-24   What is the most common type of senior abuse?

  a. caregiver neglect

  b. emotional abuse

  c. financial exploitation

  d. sexual abuse

24-25 A newly admitted 30-year old-client expresses his frustration and mounting tension related to his inability to smoke due to the No Smoking policy of the hospital. The most helpful intervention the nurse could perform would be to:

a. provide educational material regarding the dangers of smoking.

b. reveal methods the nurse himself used to quit smoking.

c. suggest diversional activities to diminish the urge to smoke.

d. request the physician to order a mild tranquilizer for the client.

24-26 The nurse recognizes that the 45-year-old client has reached Fowler's paradoxical-consolidative stage of moral development when he says,:

a. "It has taken me a long time, but I believe that Christianity is the only true faith."

b. "I believe that all faiths have a beneficial spiritual structure for their followers."

c. "Religious faith and spiritual growth is only for fools and children."

d. "I am too old and confused to know what I believe."

24-27 The nurse recognizes a teaching opportunity when her 30-year-old friend says:

a. "I don't miss a month doing my breast self-exam."

b. "I don't need to be worried about osteoporosis yet."

c. "I only get to exercise three times a week."

d. "I don't need to have a Pap smear until I am in menopause."

24-28 When a man sees his 80-year-old father struggling to clean his shotguns at the beginning of hunting season, the most supportive activity the son could do is to:

a. complete the task for him to save his father's energy.

b. confiscate the ammunition as a precaution against suicide.

c. sit with his father and compliment him on his thoroughness.

d. point out a more efficient technique to educate him.

c
Application
Analysis/Diagnosis
Psychological:
Coping and
Adaptation

24-29 While talking to the home health nurse, a 50-year-old woman who is caring for her parents who have Alzheimer's disease bursts into tears and says, "I am a total wreck. I haven't been able to sit down to eat a meal or watch a whole TV program in months." The most appropriate nursing diagnosis for this client would be:

a. Ineffective Individual Coping related to inability to meet family care needs

b. Impaired Mobility related to family care needs

c. Caregiver Role Stress related to time constraints of family care needs

d. Anxiety related to inability to meet family care needs

b
Application
Implementation
Promotion: Growth
and Development
Through the Life
Span

24-30 To enhance the maintenance of long-term memory in older adults, the nurse should encourage her older adult clients to:

a. listen to music from their youth.

b. complete crossword puzzles.

c. watch current news broadcasts.

d. care for their daily hygiene needs independently.

d
Application
Assessment
Psychosocial:
Coping and
Adaptation

24-31 Which of the following client may have a deficit in short-term memory?

a. a 70-year-old who does not remember his first grade teacher's name.

b. a 50-year-old who does not remember his lawyer's phone number even although he calls him once a month

c. a 40-year-old who does not remember his wife's birthday

d. a 60-year-old who does not remember items his wife told him to get at the store

25-1   The nurse says, "Did you sleep well last night?" The client answers, "No, I just was not sleepy." What component of the communication process does the client's response represent?

    a. sender

    b. message

    c. response/feedback

    d. decoding

25-2   The nurse says to the client, "Your M.D. is still in ICU, but he has ordered an ABG to be drawn prior to your pre-op." The nurse is risking which threat to effective communication?

    a. cultural differences

    b. language barriers

    c. encoding/decoding misinterpretations

    d. distance/space constraints

25-3   A client who is newly diagnosed with diabetes says that she knows that her illness is complicated. She says, "I wonder if I'll ever be able to completely understand it." What would be the most helpful reply by the nurse?

    a. "Have you read the pamphlets I gave you on diabetes?"

    b. "Don't worry. A lot of people have diabetes and they manage."

    c. "What is it about your illness that you don't understand?"

    d. "You should probably talk to your physician about this."

25-4   During which phase of the relationship process does clarification of the problem occur?

    a. preinteraction phase

    b. introductory phase

    c. working phase

    d. termination phase

25-5   During which phase of the relationship process are the nurse and client most likely to experience feelings of loss?

    a. preinteraction phase

    b. introductory phase

    c. working phase

    d. termination phase

c
Knowledge
Implementation
Psychosocial:
Coping and
Adaptation

25-6   During which phase of the relationship process does the nurse assist the client to explore thoughts, feelings, and actions?

a. preinteraction phase

b. introductory phase

c. working phase

d. termination phase

a
Comprehension
Implementation
Safety: Management
of Care

25-7   A client complains that his 9:00 P.M. snack was not delivered until 10:30 P.M. The nurse responds by saying that there was an emergency and she was not able to bring it in earlier. What kind of response is this?

a. defensive

b. clarifying

c. challenging

d. disagreeing

b
Application
Implementation
Psychosocial:
Coping and
Adaptation

25-8   A 45-year-old client with terminal cancer is in extreme pain and very restless. The physician wants to write a do-not-resuscitate (DNR) order, but the client's wife refuses. In order to facilitate communication with the family, it is most important for the nurse to first:

a. explain the rationale for the DNR order.

b. accept the family's wishes.

c. encourage autonomy for the client.

d. express concern about the client's possible addiction to the pain medication.

a
Application
Implementation
Safety: Management
of Care

25.9   A 50-year-old client with AIDS is receiving several IV medications and is on a cardiac monitor. The nurse comes into the room and spends five minutes regulating the IV and examining the heart monitor printout before speaking. What attitude does the nurse display?

a. coldness

b. condescension

c. insecurity

d. lack of interest

d
Application
Implementation
Psychosocial:
Coping and
Adaptation

25-10   A nurse caring for a dying client sees the client's life partner crying. In order to facilitate the discussion of feelings, the best comment she could make to the visitor would be:

a. "How are you feeling today?"

b. "You seem upset. Is your friend worse today?"

c. "Crying is good for you. Things will look brighter tomorrow."

d. "I see you have been crying. Would you like to talk about it?"

25-11 The wife of a dying client states she is overwhelmed by her husband's illness and doesn't think she can go on much longer. The nurse responds by saying, "It must be difficult having a loved one in such critical condition. Would you like to talk about it?" This is an example of:

a. focusing.

b. clarifying.

c. summarizing.

d. providing general leads.

25-12 While taking an admission history from the mother of an 18-month-old being admitted for surgery, the nurse notes that the mother is twisting her rings, running her hands through her hair, and moving about restlessly. When the nurse asks the mother about any problems or concerns, she replies, "Everything is just fine." The mother's behavior is an example of:

a. inappropriate communication.

b. inadequate language skills.

c. the violation of personal space.

d. incongruent nonverbal communication.

25-13 In order to listen attentively to a client, the nurse needs to:

a. maintain good eye contact.

b. lean back in her chair.

c. sit with her legs crossed.

d. respond quickly to the client's statements.

25.14 The nurse violates a client's personal space when he:

a. sits at the client's bedside.

b. adjusts the client's IV flow rate.

c. removes the client's abdominal sutures.

d. enters the client's hospital room.

25-15 The biggest inhibitor of effective communication is:

a. failing to listen.

b. giving false reassurance.

d. disagreeing with the client.

d. passing judgment on the client.

d
Knowledge
Evaluation
Psychosocial:
Coping and
Adaptation

25-16   One feature of an effective group is that:

a.   disagreement among members is not tolerated.

b.   the leader dominates the group.

c.   feelings are kept out of group discussions.

d.   the group is able to examine its own process.

d
Application
Implementation
Psychosocial:
Coping and
Adaptation

25-17   The client says, "I'm a failure." The nurse replies, "The plant downsized and you lost your job." The nurse is:

a.   being genuine.

b.   showing respect for the client.

c.   confronting the client.

d.   helping the client to be concrete and specific.

c
Application
Implementation
Promotion: Growth
and Development
Through the Life
Span

25-18   A few hours after the birth of her daughter, the nurse notices that the client is crying. When questioned, she says, "My husband is so disappointed in me, and I really did not want another girl either." The nurse's most therapeutic reply at this moment would be:

a.   "It is the father who determines the sex of a baby, perhaps we should tell your husband that."

b.   "It's not your fault. Don't feel bad."

c.   "You seem very upset. Would it help to talk to me about it?"

d.   "You shouldn't cry. Your baby is healthy. You can have a boy next time."

a
Comprehension
Assessment
Psychosocial:
Coping and
Adaptation

25-19   How can the nurse obtain the most accurate and truthful information about what a client is feeling when he is talking about a bad experience he has had?

a.   Observe the client's body language.

b.   Ask, "What are you feeling right now?"

c.   Ask a family member what the client is feeling.

d.   Say, "That must have been hard for you."

b
Application
Implementation
Safety: Management
of Care

25-20   While bathing a 55-year-old woman, the nurse believes she is showing warmth and caring when she says, "Turn on your side now, honey." However, the client responds in an offended tone, "My name is Mrs. Hamilton." Which factor is at work in the miscommunication that occurred?

a.   ability of the client to interpret the message

b.   different perceptions of sender and receiver

c.   incongruence between verbal and nonverbal messages

d.   lack of consideration of proxemics

a
Knowledge.
Implementation
Psychosocial:
Coping and
Adaptation

25-21 What is a small voluntary group of people who share a similar health problem (e.g., Alcoholics Anonymous)?

a. self-help group

b. teaching group

c. task group

d. self-awareness group

c
Application
Implementation
Psychosocial:
Coping and
Adaptation

25-22 A client says to the nurse, "That night nurse needs to go back to school. She gave me a shot in the wrong arm, she forgot to fill my water pitcher, and she wouldn't answer my light!" What would be a therapeutic response by the nurse?

a. "We are always understaffed on nights. I'm sure the nurse did the best she could."

b. "Well, the least competent nurses do sort of drift to the night shift. I don't blame you for being upset."

c. "Sounds like you had a bad night. Tell me more about it and lets see if there is anything I can do to help you now."

d. "You seem fine this morning. I guess it couldn't have been all that bad."

a
Application
Implementation
Safety: Management
of Care

25-23 The client tells the nurse, "I still hurt after taking two doses of my medicine. The physical therapy makes me hurt worse and the heating pad doesn't help either." Which of the following responses would enhance clarification?

a. "Are you saying that none of the therapies relieve your pain?"

b. "Perhaps the medication has not had time to work."

c. "You're saying the heating pad is not working?"

d. "Let's try changing your position in the bed."

b
Application
Evaluation
Safety: Management
of Care

25-24 Which question would be most effective in evaluating the client's understanding of teaching?

a. "Do you understand what you need to do prior to your x-ray procedure?"

b. "What do you need to do prior to your x-ray procedure?"

c. "Do you have any questions about your x-ray procedure?"

d. "Have I been clear about what you need to do prior to your x-ray procedure?"

d
Comprehension
Implementation
Physiological:
Pharmacological and
Parenteral Therapies

25-25   Which nursing intervention would meet a client's physical comfort need?

a.   responding openly about the purpose of an IV medication to establish trust

b.   accepting a client's anger and frustration about a delay in a treatment

c.   asking the client's arm preference prior to the insertion of an IV line

d.   painlessly inserting the needle for an IV medication

d
Application
Evaluation
Physiological: Basic
Care and Comfort

25-26   The nurse recognizes that a client who has constant pain from severe burns to both hands has reached Kolcaba's state of transcendence when the client is comfortable enough to:

a.   verbalize reduced pain following a pain medication.

b.   perform complex hand exercises slowly, in the same amount of time as usual.

c.   perform complex hand exercises slowly, but with ease.

d.   complete two sets of the exercises in the amount of time he previously completed first set.

d
Application
Planning
Physiological:
Pharmacological and
Parenteral Therapies

26-1   A client who is a newly diagnosed with diabetes needs to be taught about insulin injections. When would be the best time to do this teaching?

a. the day before discharge

b. when her young children are visiting

c. immediately after she is told the diagnosis

d. two days after the diagnosis when her husband is visiting

d
Comprehension
Assessment
Psychosocial:
Coping and
Adaptation

26-2   Andragogy is based on the concept that:

a. toddlers learn through imitation of their parents.

b. school-aged children learn best in brief stages because their attention spans are short.

c. adults are more motivated to learn when the material is useful to their future.

d. adults' previous experiences can be used as resources for learning.

a
Knowledge
Analysis/Diagnosis
Promotion:
Prevention and Early
Detection of Disease

26-3   When an individual experiences a need to change behavior, this is known as:

a. a learning need.

b. learning.

c. compliance.

d. differentiation.

a
Application
Implementation
Psychosocial:
Coping and
Adaptation

26-4   A nurse involved in educating a community group to appreciate the uniqueness of mentally disabled citizens is working with which domain of learning?

a. affective

b. cognitive

c. psychomotor

d. psychologic

c
Application
Evaluation
Physiological:
Physiological
Adaptation

26-5   Which of the following situations illustrates learning in the psychomotor domain?

a. The client learns the rationale for checking his heart rate prior to taking his medication.

b. The client learns the action of his cardiac medication.

c. The client learns how to palpate and count his radial pulse.

d. The client learns to accept the need for taking his medication on a daily basis.

c
Knowledge
Planning
Psychosocial:
Coping and
Adaptation

26-6　A system of activities intended to produce learning is called:

a.　cognition.

b.　objectives.

c.　teaching.

d.　readiness.

b
Knowledge
Planning
Psychosocial:
Coping and
Adaptation

26-7　Statements of measurable, desired learner behaviors are called:

a.　teaching.

b.　learning objectives.

c.　learning strategies.

d.　teaching plans.

c
Comprehension
Analysis/Diagnosis
Psychosocial:
Coping and
Adaptation

26-8　A client with diabetes who needs to learn to inject his own insulin states, "I've had a good night's sleep, so let's tackle that syringe." The client is showing which of the following?

a.　feedback

b.　active involvement

c.　readiness

d.　repetition

b
Comprehension
Evaluation
Physiological:
Pharmacological and
Parenteral Therapies

26-9　The client manipulates the syringe as the nurse verbally describes how to draw up the medication. The client is demonstrating which of the following?

a.　feedback

b.　active involvement

c.　readiness

d.　repetition

a
Comprehension
Implementation
Physiological:
Pharmacological and
Parenteral Therapies

26-10　After the client draws up his insulin, the nurse states, "You really did that well." This demonstrates:

a.　feedback

b.　active involvement

c.　readiness

d.　repetition

a
Comprehension
Implementation
Psychosocial:
Coping and
Adaptation

26-11　The nurse frowns when the client drops the syringe. This would be a display of:

a.　negative feedback

b.　positive feedback

c.　active involvement

d.　timing

26-12 At the end of a teaching session, the nurse suggests that the client practice drawing up and injecting medication several times before their next teaching session. This suggestion is based on the principle that:

a. readiness is essential for learning.

b. meaningful feedback enhances learning.

c. repetition facilitates retention of newly learned material.

d. learning is facilitated by organizing material so that it proceeds from simple to complex.

26-13 Which of the following best demonstrates positive reinforcement (positive feedback)?

a. A child is told he cannot watch a favorite television program because he did not follow the rules.

b. A nurse praises the client for keeping an accurate fluid intake record.

c. The nurse frowns when a client drops his insulin syringe.

d. The nurse points out errors a client makes in putting on sterile gloves.

26-14 Which of the following nursing diagnoses pertains to a client's learning needs?

a. Noncompliance with Medical Treatment related to low income

b. Altered Health Maintenance related to knowledge deficit: catheter care

c. Total Self-Care Deficit related to altered level of consciousness

d. Anxiety related to wife's illness

26-15 What is one advantage of using computer-assisted instruction (CAI)?

a. Clients can learn at the pace that suits them best.

b. The nurse-client relationship is strengthened.

c. Psychomotor skills do not need to be practiced on the actual equipment.

d. The nurse does not need to be involved in the teaching.

26-16 A written test is best for evaluating which type of learning?

a. affective

b. cognitive

c. psychomotor

d. task-oriented

a
Knowledge
Evaluation
Safety: Management
of Care

26-17   What is a reason why a nurse would use the SMOG index?

a.   readability level of teaching materials

b.   client's educational level

c.   client's cognitive ability

d.   effectiveness of the teaching

c
Comprehension
Implementation
Safety: Management
of Care

26-18   How can you simplify client educational materials and make them easier to read?

a.   Use longer sentences to ensure thorough explanations .

b.   Use technical and medical terms to reduce confusion.

c.   Use smaller words that are simple and common.

d.   Use only words that are found in current journals.

c
Knowledge
Implementation
Psychosocial:
Coping and
Adaptation

26-19   Which teaching strategy would be most effective for achieving a goal in the affective domain?

a.   providing explanations or descriptions

b.   answering questions

c.   role playing

d.   demonstrating

d
Knowledge
Evaluation
Promotion:
Prevention and Early
Detection of Disease

26-20   During which phase of the teaching process would the nurse measure client learning?

a.   assessment

b.   planning

c.   implementation

d.   evaluation

a
Comprehension
Implementation
Safety: Management
of Care

26-21   Which factor has increased the need for health teaching by nurses?

a.   shorter hospital stays

b.   emphasis on treatment rather than prevention

c.   an increase in long-term illnesses

d.   a younger population

d
Application
Implementation
Psychosocial:
Coping and
Adaptation

26-22   The nurse who wants to use a humanism approach to teaching would:

a.   design the learning objectives based on nursing assessments.

b.   carefully arrange the teaching plan to go from the simple to the complex.

c.   state learning objectives in clear, concise language.

d.   coordinate the learning objectives with the learner.

26-23   A 30-year-old female client who needs to be taught 10 stretching exercises for her burned hands says, "I'm afraid I will stretch my hands too far and ruin the skin grafts." The alert nurse will alter the teaching plan to:

   a.   teach only the first five simple exercises first to lessen anxiety.

   b.   demonstrate all 15 exercises prior to starting instruction on each individual exercise.

   c.   lead the client through stretches slowly, requesting constant feedback about discomfort.

   d.   request that the physician speak with the client to lessen her anxiety.

26-24   Which of the following nursing actions facilitates learning?

   a.   Request that the parents of a four-year-old boy participate in the instruction on using a medicated mouthwash.

   b.   Instruct a 16-year-old girl in complex hand exercises during a time when the parents are absent.

   c.   Arrange for a 50-year-old female nurse to instruct a 14-year-old boy in self-urinary catheterization.

   d.   Let a 70-year-old client perform the colostomy irrigation procedure after watching a video.

LEADING, MANAGING, AND INFLUENCING CHANGE

c
Application
Implementation
Safety: Management
of Care

27-1 A nurse manager's transactional leadership approach is demonstrated when the manager:

a. leads the group to meet objectives through the use of the faith the group has in him.

b. supports the group to share the vision of the goal and take on leadership responsibility to meet it.

c. offers a reward or incentive to enhance the individual group members' commitment to meet the goal.

d. coordinates the combined influence of organizations within the community and other departments in the hospital to meet the goal.

a
Comprehension
Safety: Management
of Care

27-2 Which of the following is the best example of a management function?

a. directing and evaluating nursing staff members

b. influencing the decision of an ethics committee

c. explaining medication side effects to a client

d. writing a letter to the editor of a nursing journal

a
Application
Analysis
Safety: Management
of Care

27-3 A nurse identifies a better way to instruct clients with diabetes how to give themselves insulin and decides that a change is needed in the unit's diabetic teaching program. Which stage of Lewin's change theory does this represent?

a. unfreezing

b. moving

c. refreezing

d. confirmation

a
Knowledge
Safety: Management
of Care

27-4 A leader who believes that group members are incapable of making their own decisions is demonstrating:

a. autocratic leadership.

b. democratic leadership.

c. laissez-faire leadership.

d. managerial leadership.

27-5 Which style of situational leadership is demonstrated by a leader who is helping the nursing staff adopt a new computer system with which they have had no experience?

a. high task-high relationship

b. high task-low relationship

c. low task-high relationship

d. low task-low relationship

27-6 Which of the following illustrates a health care team guided by the principles of participative leadership?

a. The physician makes all decisions regarding the client's care.

b. The team utilizes the expertise of its members to influence decisions regarding the client's care.

c. Each member of the team independently makes decisions regarding the client's care without consulting the other members.

d. Nurses decide nursing care; physicians decide medical and other treatments.

27-7 In which type of leadership is empowerment of the followers an important concept?

a. laissez faire or nondirective leadership

b. autocratic leadership

c. democratic leadership

d. transformational leadership

27-8 A nurse manager's job description states that her work includes approving work schedules and directing and evaluating the work of staff nurses. This is an example of:

a. authority.

b. accountability.

c. delegation.

d. responsibility.

27-9 After making a medication error the nurse notifies the physician and completes an incident report. This is an example of:

a. authority.

b. accountability.

c. delegation.

d. democratic leadership.

c
Comprehension
Implementation
Safety: Management
of Care

27-10 When delegating aspects of a client's care to unlicensed staff members, the nurse:

a. is relieved of the need to supervise or evaluate the staff members.

b. must know how to perform the task that has been delegated.

c. is assigning the responsibility but not the accountability for those tasks.

d. should make assignments based the learning needs of the staff members.

d
Knowledge
Safety: Management
of Care

27-11 An experienced nurse who voluntarily develops a relationship with a younger, less experienced nurse with the intent of promoting her/his growth and professional advancement is called a:

a. change agent.

b. nurse manager.

c. team leader.

d. mentor.

c
Application
Safety: Management
of Care

27-12 A male staff nurse with no authority over other nurses, but who is liked and respected, uses his influence to persuade other nurses to strike for better staffing and client care conditions. He is functioning as a(n):

a. nurse manager.

b. formal leader.

c. informal leader.

d. external change agent.

a
Application
Safety: Management
of Care

27-13 Which is an example of situational or natural change?

a. Since the onset of her child's illness, a nurse has been working night shift full-time.

b. After considering alternatives, a hospital installs a new computer system.

c. After working with a preceptor, a new graduate begins to care for her clients on her own.

d. Nurses are notified that they may no longer park in the covered parking area effective immediately.

a
Application
Safety: Management
of Care

27-14 The nurse manager realizes that working with the new computer system will be stressful for the staff nurses. She is aware that they do not view this change positively. She hopes to help them survive the stress of change by:

a. providing opportunities for them to talk about the system and provide support for each other.

b. convincing them that it is beyond their control anyway, so it is best to just accept it.

c. acknowledging that they do not value the change and reassuring them that this does not matter.

d. letting individual nurses decide whether they want to use the computers or continue charting in the old way.

c
Application
Implementation
Safety: Management
of Care

27-15 A new computer system has been installed and two of the nurses have been putting up serious resistance by complaining to other nurses and reporting computer failure, among other actions. Which action by the nurse manager might be helpful in dealing with their resistance?

a. Maintain a climate of discipline by explaining that griping and complaining are not helpful.

b. Avoid these nurses and ignore their resistance until the problem blows over.

c. Talk to the two nurses and find out the reasons for their opposition to the new system.

d. Admit the system is not perfect and reveal that she also has had second thoughts about it.

a
Application
Safety: Management
of Care

27-16 A certain male oncology clinical nurse specialist does not direct or evaluate the work of the staff nurses nor have the authority to enforce decisions about nursing care, but he is respected for his knowledge and ability and has a great deal of influence. He has instituted a number of changes in the nursing care on the oncology unit. What type of power does he have?

a. expert power

b. reward power

c. legitimate power

d. transformative power

d
Application
Safety: Management
of Care

27-17 Which nurse is demonstrating a characteristic of an effective manager?

a. Bob, who aggressively attacks all situations in need of change to express his autonomy

b. Tessa, who knows how to agitate the administration to get their attention and doesn't hesitate to do it

c. Kent, who avoids using a mentor because he believes it would compromise his ability to make fair decisions

d. Althea, who uses written and oral communication skills to express herself clearly and effectively

a
Application
Assessment
Safety: Management
of Care

27-18 A nurse manager has introduced a new computer system to track inservice hours, but it has met with resistance from the staff. Which of these staff members is most advanced in their acceptance of the change?

a. Joe, who tried it out but still feels that is time consuming

b. Ann, who asks more about the system

c. Sue who says, "I don't see how it is any better than what we are doing now."

d. Bill who says, "I just found out about the new system. It sounds great!"

b
Application
Safety: Management
of Care

27-19 The nurse manager who selects the situational leadership style of delegation to approach a change in the care of clients with decubitis ulcers must have a group that is:

a. willing but lacking in experience.

b. competent and willing.

c. able but resistant.

d. lacking in experience and resistant.

b
Application
Safety: Management
of Care

27-20 Having accepted the need to change the system of staff rotation, the nurse manager collects data about alternate rotation plans, sends out surveys to staff members, and selects an optimum time to initiate the new rotation. The nurse manager is demonstrating which level in Lewin's change model?

a. unfreezing

b. moving

c. refreezing

d. transformation

27-21 A group of staff nurses approach the nurse manager about their discontent with the current dress code. The bureaucratic nurse manager would:

a. ask the group to bring their ideas for change with all their supporting data to the next staff meeting.

b. calmly explain that the dress code policy is set by the institution and the administration at the annual meeting and is enforced by the human resources department.

c. sit down with the group and facilitate their process to make change by offering information and constructive criticism.

d. direct the group to write a request to wear any color of scrubs and type of athletic shoe they desire.

27-22 When a nurse manager evaluates the performance of a staff member and helps organize a plan of improved performance, the manager is acting in which managing role?

a. planning

b. organizing

c. directing

d. controlling

a
Comprehension
Assessment
Promotion: Growth
and Development
Through the Life
Span

28-1 Body temperature is the balance between heat production and heat loss. Which of the following healthy individuals would probably have the highest body temperature?

   a.   a 16-year-old boy who just walked 2 miles

   b.   a 16-year-old boy who is watching television

   c.   a 65-year-old man who just walked 2 miles

   d.   a 65-year-old man who is watching television

c
Comprehension
Assessment
Promotion:
Prevention and Early
Detection of Disease

28-2 An oral temperature would be contraindicated for a client who:

   a.   has a high fever.

   b.   is going to surgery in the next hour.

   c.   is confused.

   d.   has a severe cardiac problem.

c
Knowledge
Assessment
Physiological:
Physiological
Adaptation

28-3 Which of the following factors influences the body's heat production?

   a.   protein intake

   b.   diaphragmatic breathing

   c.   sympathetic stimulation

   d.   sweating

d
Knowledge
Physiological:
Physiological
Adaptation

28-4 Insensible heat loss occurs through the mechanism of:

   a.   radiation.

   b.   conduction.

   c.   convection.

   d.   vaporization.

b
Comprehension
Analysis
Physiological:
Physiological
Adaptation

28-5 During the past 24 hours, a client's temperature has fluctuated widely above the normal range. The nurse should record this as a(n):

   a.   intermittent fever.

   b.   remittent fever.

   c.   relapsing fever.

   d.   constant fever.

c
Knowledge
Assessment
Promotion:
Prevention and Early
Detection of Disease

28-6 To obtain an accurate reading using the axillary route, the nurse must leave the thermometer in place for:

   a.   2 minutes.

   b.   3 minutes.

   c.   9 minutes.

   d.   15 minutes.

a Application Analysis Physiological: Physiological Adaptation	28-7	A 2-year-old client with a medical diagnosis of intestinal virus has a rectal temperature of 102.8° F. She says she is cold. She has been vomiting for the past two days. An appropriate nursing diagnosis would be: a. Hyperthermia related to dehydration. b. Hyperthermia related to excess heat production. c. Hyperthermia related to environmental temperature. d. Hypothermia related to vomiting.
c Application Implementation Physiological: Physiological Adaptation	28-8	A 2-year-old client who has a rectal temperature of 102.8° F begins to sweat profusely. Because she is in the flush phase of her fever, the appropriate action for the nurse would be to: a. apply ice packs to axilla and groin. b. increase her physical activity. c. give her a tepid sponge bath. d. provide extra blankets.
c Knowledge Assessment Promotion: Growth and Development Through the Life Span	28-9	What is the average resting heart rate for a two-year-old child? a. 60 bpm b. 80 bpm c. 110 bpm d. 160 bpm
a Knowledge Assessment Promotion: Prevention and Early Detection of Disease	28-10	What is the appropriate site for taking the pulse of a normal two-year-old child? a. apical b. radial c. brachial d. temporal
d Knowledge Assessment Promotion: Prevention and Early Detection of Disease	28-11	The thumb is not used in palpating a pulse because: a. the index finger is more sensitive to touch. b. thumb pressure may obliterate the pulse. c. it is more awkward. d. the nurse might feel his/her own thumb pulse.
c Knowledge Assessment Promotion: Prevention and Early Detection of Disease	28-12	In an adult, the apex of the heart is located: a. left of the sternum at the 2nd intercostal space. b. right of the sternum at the 3rd intercostal space. c. left of the sternum and under the 4th, 5th, or 6th intercostal space. d. right of the sternum and under the 4th, 5th, or 6th intercostal space.

28-13 A 40-year-old client with fractures of both arms has bilateral casts from his shoulders to his hands. Which of the following is the best method of obtaining and monitoring his pulse?

a. take his temporal pulse

b. place the client on a cardiac monitor

c. omit taking the pulse if his other vital signs are normal

d. inform the physician that the pulse cannot be monitored

28-14 For a 40-year-old male, which of the following sets of vital signs would be considered normal?

a. BP 130/72, pulse 73, respirations 16

b. BP 90/60, pulse 70, respirations 32

c. BP 100/50, pulse 44, respirations 10

d. BP 180/100, pulse 72, respirations 20

28-15 As you begin to take a client's oral temperature, she tells you that she has just had some ice chips. The appropriate nursing action is to:

a. give her a sip of warm water, wait five minutes, then take her temperature.

b. take a rectal temperature.

c. proceed to take the oral temperature.

d. wait 30 minutes before taking an oral temperature.

28-16 The interchange of oxygen and carbon dioxide between the alveoli of the lungs and the pulmonary blood is called:

a. external respiration.

b. internal respiration.

c. inspiration.

d. ventilation.

28-17 Normal breathing rate is referred to as:

a. apnea.

b. bradypnea.

c. eupnea.

d. tachypnea.

28-18 The diastolic blood pressure is:

a. the result of the contraction of the ventricles.

b. a reflection of changes in cardiac output.

c. the minimum pressure present at all times within the arteries.

d. an average of the systolic pressure and the pulse pressure.

b
Comprehension
Assessment
Physiological:
Physiological
Adaptation

28-19   It is especially important to watch for a decrease in blood pressure in a
         client who:

a.   is obese.

b.   is hemorrhaging.

c.   has a fever.

d.   has been exposed to cold temperatures.

a
Knowledge
Assessment
Promotion:
Prevention and Early
Detection of Disease

28-20   When measuring blood pressure, the first sound you hear on release of
         the valve indicates the:

a.   systolic pressure.

b.   diastolic pressure.

c.   pulse pressure.

d.   auscultatory gap.

b
Comprehension
Assessment
Promotion:
Prevention and Early
Detection of Disease

28-21   In a blood pressure reading of 120/90, the 90 reflects the:

a.   pressure present in arteries during contraction of heart ventricles.

b.   pressure present in arteries while ventricles are at rest.

c.   difference between systolic and diastolic pressure.

d.   pulse pressure.

d
Application
Assessment
Promotion:
Prevention and Early
Detection of Disease

28-22   Which of the following healthy clients would you expect to have the
         highest blood pressure?

a.   a 40-year-old obese Anglo-American female

b.   a 40-year-old Anglo-American male of normal weight

c.   a 60-year-old African-American male of normal weight

d.   a 60-year-old obese African-American male

c
Application
Assessment
Promotion:
Prevention and Early
Detection of Disease

28-23   Which method should the nurse use to obtain the blood pressure of a
         client with both a known auscultatory gap and a peripheral circulation
         problem?

a.   auscultatory method in the non-dominant arm

b.   auscultatory method in the thigh

c.   palpatory method in either arm

d.   flush method in either arm

a
Comprehension
Analysis
Physiological:
Physiological
Adaptation

28-24   A client has a temperature of 101° F and is shivering and complaining
         that he is cold. Which of the following symptoms would help to confirm
         that the fever is in the onset stage?

a.   pale, cold skin

b.   flushed, warm

c.   increased thirst

d.   sweating

28-25 Which of the following is a risk factor for hypothermia?

a. alcoholism

b. infection

c. central nervous system disease

d. head trauma

28-26 Many agencies use electronic tympanic membrane thermometers. Which of the following is true regarding their use?

a. Repeated measurements are very consistent.

b. Results are obtained very quickly.

c. Readings are more accurate than rectal temperatures.

d. It is a completely safe procedure.

28-27 The nurse is unable to palpate the client's popliteal pulse. Presence of which of the following pulses indicates adequate popliteal artery flow?

a. femoral

b. pedal

c. brachial

d. carotid

28-28 While releasing the blood pressure cuff below the systolic reading, the nurse is uncertain exactly where the sound becomes muffled. What would be the best action for the nurse to take?

a. Before releasing the cuff completely, immediately pump the cuff back up and begin lowering again.

b. Release the cuff completely, wait one to two minutes, and retake the entire blood pressure.

c. Ask another nurse to take the blood pressure, and compare the two readings.

d. Take the blood pressure on the client's other arm.

c
Application
Assessment
Psychosocial:
Coping and
Adaptation

29-1   A client is somewhat hesitant to respond during an interview and the nurse decides that further psychologic assessment is indicated. In order to assess the client's mood, the nurse should begin by asking her:

    a.   how she usually copes with stress.

    b.   what major stressors she has experienced in the past year.

    c.   if she feels down or cries frequently.

    d.   if she has ever tried to kill herself.

a
Knowledge
Assessment
Promotion:
Prevention and Early
Detection of Disease

29-2   Which one of the following entries found in a client's record probably comes from the nursing health history?

    a.   no known allergies

    b.   blood pressure 130/84

    c.   skin dry and pale

    d.   able to repeat seven digits without error

b
Comprehension
Assessment
Promotion:
Prevention and Early
Detection of Disease

29-3   When obtaining the nursing health history on a client with a medical diagnosis of pneumonia, which of the following questions would best elicit his chief complaint?

    a.   "How would you describe your health up to this time?"

    b.   "What caused you to come to the hospital?"

    c.   "Have you been hospitalized for this problem in the past?"

    d.   "Has anyone in your family ever had pneumonia?"

a
Knowledge
Assessment
Promotion:
Prevention and Early
Detection of Disease

29-4   In which part of the nursing health history would you find information about a client's immunizations?

    a.   past history

    b.   review of systems

    c.   lifestyle data

    d.   biographic data

b
Comprehension
Planning
Promotion:
Prevention and Early
Detection of Disease

29-5   Information from a client's educational history can help the nurse to:

    a.   understand the client's customs and beliefs.

    b.   make appropriate adjustments in plans for client teaching.

    c.   assess whether the client has a support system at home.

    d.   determine the client's financial status.

d
Comprehension
Assessment
Promotion:
Prevention and Early
Detection of Disease

29-6   One of the purposes of a physical health examination is to:

a.   elicit information about all the variables that may affect the client's health status.

b.   obtain data that will help the nurse understand and appreciate the client's life experiences.

c.   initiate a nonjudgmental, trusting, interpersonal relationship with the client.

d.   evaluate the physiologic outcomes of health care and thus the progress of a client's health problem.

c
Application
Implementation
Promotion:
Prevention and Early
Detection of Disease

29-7   When preparing a client for a physical health examination, the nurse should:

a.   omit draping in order to have the client's entire body accessible.

b.   ensure that a consent form has been signed.

c.   explain the purpose of the exam and what to expect.

d.   have the client drink water in order to fill the bladder.

b
Knowledge
Assessment
Promotion:
Prevention and Early
Detection of Disease

29-8   A client is in a side-lying position with the lower arm positioned behind her head, the upper arm flexed at the shoulder and elbow, and both legs flexed in front of the body. What position is this?

a.   lithotomy

b.   Sims'

c.   horizontal recumbent

d.   dorsal recumbent

a
Knowledge
Assessment
Promotion:
Prevention and Early
Detection of Disease

29-9   What position would be best for conducting a vaginal examination?

a.   lithotomy

b.   Sims'

c.   genupectoral (knee-chest)

d.   dorsal recumbent

A
Knowledge
Assessment
Promotion:
Prevention and Early
Detection of Disease

29-10   The technique in which the nurse listens to sounds produced in the body is called:

a.   auscultation.

b.   inspection.

c.   palpation.

d.   percussion.

b
Knowledge
Assessment
Promotion:
Prevention and Early
Detection of Disease

29-11   Data concerning the client's overall appearance and behavior are part of
the:

a.   review of systems.

b.   general survey.

c.   physical health examination.

d.   focused assessment.

a
Knowledge
Assessment
Promotion:
Prevention and Early
Detection of Disease

29-12   As a part of the general survey, the nurse collects data about the client's:

a.   height and weight.

b.   skin turgor.

c.   pupillary reflexes.

d.   breath sounds.

c
Knowledge
Assessment
Physiological:
Reduction of Risk
Potential

29-13   The Glasgow Coma Scale is used to assess a client's:

a.   mood.

b.   musculoskeletal status.

c.   neurological status.

d.   communication ability.

d
Application
Assessment
Physiological:
Reduction of Risk
Potential

29-14   To assess a client's level of consciousness, the nurse should:

a.   ask the client to recite the alphabet.

b.   have the client identify common objects in the room.

c.   test the client's Achilles reflex.

d.   ask the client to move a part of his/her body.

a
Knowledge
Analysis
Physiological: Basic
Care and Comfort

29-15   Skin turgor is a measurement of:

a.   hydration.

b.   strength.

c.   motor function.

d.   pain.

b
Knowledge
Assessment
Promotion:
Prevention and Early
Detection of Disease

29-16   When auscultating the heart of a normal adult, how many heart sounds
should the nurse expect to hear?

a.   one

b.   two

c.   three

d.   four

a
Knowledge
Assessment
Physiological:
Reduction of Risk
Potential

29-17 The blanch test is done to assess:

a. peripheral circulation.

b. edema.

c. pain.

d. skin temperature.

d
Knowledge
Analysis
Physiological:
Physiological
Adaptation

29-18 A barrel chest is generally seen in clients with:

a. congenital skeletal defect.

b. obesity.

c. excessive muscular development.

d. emphysema (lung disease).

b
Comprehension
Analysis
Physiological:
Reduction of Risk
Potential

29-19 The nurse asked the client to dorsiflex her foot. Upon doing so, the client gasped and said, "That really hurt." The nurse should recognize this as a:

a. contracture.

b. positive Homan's sign.

c. positive Romberg's sign.

d. muscle cramp.

b
Knowledge
Assessment
Promotion:
Prevention and Early
Detection of Disease

29-20 Which techniques of abdominal assessment should one definitely expect beginning practitioners to perform competently?

a. auscultation and percussion

b. auscultation and inspection

c. inspection and palpation

d. palpation and percussion

c
Knowledge
Assessment
Promotion:
Prevention and Early
Detection of Disease

29-21 When auscultating for bowel sounds, approximately how long must the nurse listen before concluding that bowel sounds are absent?

a. 30 to 60 seconds

b. 1 to 2 minutes

c. 3 to 5 minutes

d. 10 to 15 minutes

c
Knowledge
Assessment
Promotion:
Prevention and Early
Detection of Disease

29-22 Where in the abdomen is the stomach located?

a. right upper quadrant

b. right lower quadrant

c. left upper quadrant

d. left lower quadrant

c
Knowledge
Assessment
Physiological:
Physiological
Adaptation

29-23   The term *alopecia* means:

    a.   inequality of pupil diameters.

    b.   a gurgling sound heard over the large intestine.

    c.   baldness or deficiency of hair.

    d.   offensive sweat found mostly in the axillae.

b
Comprehension
Assessment
Promotion:
Prevention and Early
Detection of Disease

29-24   Which of the following is a normal finding when examining the nails?

    a.   koilonychia

    b.   colorless, convex nail plate

    c.   thin, grooved nails

    d.   angle between nail and nail bed greater than 180 degrees

d
Knowledge
Analysis
Physiological:
Physiological
Adaptation

29-25   An acute or chronic infection of the marginal structures of a finger or toe nail is called:

    a.   stereognosis.

    b.   hordeolum.

    c.   mydriasis.

    d.   paronychia.

b
Application
Implementation
Physiological:
Physiological
Adaptation

29-26   When palpating the client's abdomen, the nurse thinks he feels an inguinal hernia. The nurse should:

    a.   call the physician as soon as possible.

    b.   ask the client to raise his head and shoulders from the pillow without using his arms for support.

    c.   stop palpating and return later when the client's bladder has filled.

    d.   ask the client to take a deep breath and hold it while he palpates again.

a
Knowledge
Assessment
Promotion: Growth
and Development
Through the Life
Span

29-27   Which of the following musculoskeletal changes is commonly seen in the older client?

    a.   decreased coordination

    b.   loss of Achilles reflex

    c.   positive Romberg's sign

    d.   increased bone mass

a
Knowledge
Assessment
Promotion: Growth
and Development
Through the Life
Span

29-28 Which of the following physical changes occur in the eyes of the older client?

a. Visual acuity is decreased as the lenses becomes more opaque and lose elasticity.

b. Eyes appear watery due to the increase in tear production.

c. Pupils' reaction to light and accommodation become asymmetrical.

d. Peripheral vision increases due to the ability of the iris to accommodate.

c
Knowledge
Assessment
Promotion: Growth
and Development
Through the Life
Span

29-29 When assessing an older client's thorax and breathing patterns, which of the following is a normal finding?

a. an increased depth of respiration

b. an increase in respiratory rate at rest

c. a barrel-chested appearance

d. use of accessory muscles during inspiration

d
Knowledge
Analysis
Physiological:
Physiological
Adaptation

29-30 When assessing a client's skin, the nurse observes small, slightly red, raised, solid lesions less than 1 cm in size. They appear to be pimples, but are not pus-filled. In the health assessment, the nurse should describe these lesions as:

a. macules.

b. nodules.

c. vesicles.

d. papules.

a
Comprehension
Assessment
Promotion: Growth
and Development
Through the Life
Span

29-31 When assessing children, which one of the following should be left for the end portion of the exam?

a. abdomen

b. heart

c. face

d. legs

C
Comprehension
Assessment
Promotion:
Prevention and Early
Detection of Disease

29-32 When percussing over normal lung tissue, the nurse should hear sounds that are:

a. flat, soft, high-pitched.

b. dull, medium loud, medium-pitched.

c. resonant, loud, low-pitched.

d. tympanic, very loud, high-pitched.

a
Knowledge
Assessment
Promotion:
Prevention and Early
Detection of Disease

29-33 To assess physical fitness, which parameter should the nurse check to attain the recovery index?

a. heart rate

b. blood pressure

c. respiratory rate

d. vital capacity

b
Knowledge
Assessment
Promotion:
Prevention and Early
Detection of Disease

29-34 The nurse hears adventitious sounds in the right midclavicular line at the level of the 6th rib. This location reflects the:

a. right upper lobe

b. right middle lobe

c. right lower lobe

d. mediastinum

d
Application
Assessment
Promotion: Growth
and Development
Through the Life
Span

29-35 A 14-month-old child has been walking for two months. Which assessment finding is normal?

a. asymmetry of the legs

b. scoliosis

c. dorsiflexion of feet

d. bow legs

c
Application
Assessment
Promotion:
Prevention and Early
Detection of Disease

29-36 Which cranial nerve is the nurse testing when she asks the client to clench his teeth?

a. facial

b. hypoglossal

c. trigeminal

d. trochlear

b
Application
Diagnosis
Physiological:
Physiological
Adaptation

29-37 The nurse is writing a diagnosis for a client with wheezing. Which nursing diagnosis is appropriate?

a. Altered Tissue Perfusion related to slowed circulation

b. Ineffective Airway Clearance related to increased secretions

c. Anxiety related to fear of hospitals

d. Social Isolation related to chronic disease

b
Application
Implementation
Physiological: Basic
Care and Comfort

29-38 During a physical exam, the nurse notes the client has red, swollen gums. The client states the gums bleed occasionally. The nurse documents this as:

a. plaque along the gums.

b. peridontal disease.

c. acute stomatitis.

d. chronic sores.

c
Comprehension
Implementation
Safety: Safety and
Infection Control

30-1 When caring for a client with AIDS-related cancer, the nurse should always use which of the following protective measures?

a. gloves, gown, and mask

b. gloves

c. standard precautions

d. no precautions

a
Knowledge
Safety: Safety and
Infection Control

30-2 In the United States, which is the primary public health agency concerned with disease prevention, tracking and management of infectious diseases at the national level?

a. Centers for Disease Control and Prevention

b. World Health Organization

c. Department of Health and Human Services

d. National Institute for Occupational Safety and Health

c
Knowledge
Physiological:
Physiological
Adaptation

30-3 Which of the following is an example of a nonspecific body defense against infection?

a. cellular immunity

b. antibodies

c. inflammatory response

d. phagocytes

c
Comprehension
Assessment
Physiological:
Physiological
Adaptation

30-4 An entry in the client's chart describes wound drainage as 'sanguineous'. This means that it:

a. is watery in appearance.

b. varies in color (either green-tinged or yellow).

c. contains large amounts of red blood cells.

d. is foul smelling and comprised chiefly of serum.

a
Knowledge
Physiological:
Physiological
Adaptation

30-5 Of the following bodily defenses against infection, which one is an example of a specific defense?

a. lymphocyte formation

b. intact skin

c. nasal cilia

d. stomach acid

c
Knowledge
Analysis
Physiological:
Physiological
Adaptation

30-6   A client has an inflammatory response to an infection. The involved area is swollen and bruised and has yellow drainage and pus-filled lesions. Which of these clinical findings is a cardinal sign of the inflammatory response?

    a.   yellow drainage

    b.   pus-filled lesions

    c.   swelling

    d.   bruising

a
Knowledge
Physiological:
Physiological
Adaptation

30-7   A foreign protein that invades the body is called a(n):

    a.   antigen.

    b.   interferon.

    c.   complement.

    d.   antibody.

d
Comprehension
Physiological:
Physiological
Adaptation

30-8   Which of the following best describes *humoral immunity*?

    a.   It is mediated by the T-cell system.

    b.   It primarily defends against fungal infections.

    c.   It aids in the production of lymphokines.

    d.   It is mediated by antibodies produced by B-lymphocytes.

c
Knowledge
Assessment
Physiological:
Physiological
Adaptation

30-9   Immunity obtained as a result of experiencing an illness is known as:

    a.   active natural immunity.

    b.   passive natural immunity.

    c.   active acquired immunity.

    d.   passive acquired immunity.

a
Application
Analysis
Safety: Safety and
Infection Control

30-10   As a result of sharing a needle with an HIV-positive person (Person A), Person B becomes infected. In the chain of infection, before Person B became infected, the *reservoir* was:

    a.   Person A.

    b.   Person B.

    c.   the dirty needle.

    d.   the hole made by inserting the needle into Person B's skin.

a
Application
Analysis
Safety: Safety and
Infection Control

30-11   As a result of sharing a needle with an HIV-positive person (Person A), Person B becomes infected. In the chain of infection, before Person B became infected, the *portal of exit* for the virus was:

    a.   Person A's needle puncture site.

    b.   Person B's needle puncture site.

    c.   Person A's blood.

    d.   the needle.

d
Application
Analysis
Safety: Safety and
Infection Control

30-12 As a result of sharing a needle with an HIV-positive person (Person A), Person B becomes infected. In the chain of infection, Person B was infected by indirect transmission. The *vector* (or vehicle) for transmitting the virus was:

    a. Person A's blood.

    b. Person B's blood.

    c. Person B's needle puncture site.

    d. the needle.

c
Comprehension
Assessment
Safety: Safety and
Infection Control

30-13 Which of the following situations is an example of microorganism transmission via droplet contact?

    a. Infected wound drainage contacts the nurse's hands.

    b. A virus is transmitted through sexual intercourse.

    c. Microorganisms contact a person's nasal mucous when someone coughs nearby.

    d. A contaminated stethoscope touches the skin of a client.

a
Application
Assessment
Safety: Safety and
Infection Control

30-14 Microorganisms are transmitted to a client when a contaminated stethoscope touches his skin. The stethoscope is a:

    a. vector (vehicle).

    b. portal of exit.

    c. portal of entry.

    d. reservoir.

d
Knowledge
Assessment
Safety: Safety and
Infection Control

30-15 An individual who is more likely than others to acquire an infection is a(n):

    a. etiologic agent.

    b. vehicle.

    c. reservoir.

    d. susceptible host.

d
Knowledge
Assessment
Promotion: Growth
and Development
Through the Life
Span

30-16 Which of the following groups of individuals is most susceptible to infection?

    a. middle-aged adults

    b. young adults

    c. young children

    d. newborn infants

30-17 The time when the microorganism adapts to the person and multiplies sufficiently to produce an infection is termed the:

a. incubation period.

b. prodromal period.

c. illness period.

d. convalescent period.

30-18 Which of the following situations is an example of a nosocomial infection?

a. A urinary tract infection develops in a paralyzed client who voids without catheterization.

b. A debilitated client contracts influenza from a roommate.

c. An infection develops at an intravenous infusion site because of poor insertion technique.

d. A hospitalized child develops chicken pox lesions one day after admission.

30-19 Which of the following client statements indicates a client who is at highest risk for infection?

a. "I am just about five pounds overweight according to those insurance charts."

b. "I had my last dose of chemotherapy two weeks ago, and I'm glad that's over."

c. "My life is pretty uneven right now; I'm really busy."

d. "I haven't had anything more serious than a cold in the past two years."

30-20 Of the following laboratory data, which is most indicative of infection?

a. 4,500 leukocytes/cu mm

b. 90% neutrophils

c. 4% eosinophils

d. negative blood culture

30-21 Which nurse is practicing good asepsis?

a. One who changes intravenous tubing only when the IV infiltrates or stops running.

b. One who places the urinary drainage bag on the bed while changing the linen.

c. One who wears gloves when suctioning an airway.

d. One who places a used bandage in the bedside waste basket.

b
Knowledge
Implementation
Safety: Safety and
Infection Control

30-22 Surgical asepsis differs from medical asepsis in that surgical asepsis:

    a. confines a specific microorganism to a specific area.

    b. keeps an area or object free from all microorganisms.

    c. keeps an area or object free from pathogens.

    d. limits the number of microorganisms in an area.

b
Comprehension
Implementation
Safety: Safety and
Infection Control

30-23 Which of the following situations has the highest potential for contaminating a sterile field?

    a. The nurse diverts her head from the sterile field when talking.

    b. The nurse turns her back on the sterile field.

    c. The nurse holds her sterile gloved hands above waist level.

    d. The nurse reaches around a sterile field.

d
Application
Implementation
Safety: Safety and
Infection Control

30-24 The nurse is inserting an intravenous catheter. Which statement by the nurse would provide the client with the most knowledge about his need to maintain sterile technique during the procedure?

    a. "Don't move because you could cause the needle to move out of the vein."

    b. "I'll be wearing sterile gloves while I insert your IV"

    c. "Keep your head turned to the right while I insert this IV catheter."

    d. "Try not to cough because germs from your lungs could contaminate the IV insertion site."

a
Knowledge
Implementation
Safety: Safety and
Infection Control

30-25 For routine client care, the Centers for Disease Control and Prevention recommend vigorous hand washing under a stream of water for at least:

    a. 10 seconds.

    b. 30 seconds.

    c. 1 minute.

    d. 2 minutes.

c
Knowledge
Implementation
Safety: Safety and
Infection Control

30-26 Which of the following category-specific isolation precautions requires that gowns, masks, and gloves be worn by all persons entering the room?

    a. contact isolation

    b. enteric precautions

    c. strict isolation

    d. universal precautions

a
Application
Planning
Safety: Safety and
Infection Control

30-27 Which of the following clients most requires a private room?

    a. a client who has hepatitis B and is incontinent

    b. a client who has an infected abdominal incision

    c. a client who has a kidney infection

    d. a client who is bedfast and has an infected decubitus ulcer

b
Application
Implementation
Safety: Safety and
Infection Control

30-28   If the nurse is wearing gloves, gown, and mask, which item should be removed first when preparing to exit the client's room?

a.   gown

b.   gloves

c.   mask

d.   the order is not important

a
Application
Evaluation
Safety: Safety and
Infection Control

30-29   The nurse would know that proper teaching of transmission-based precautions in a hospital has been accomplished if visitors for a client with tuberculosis:

a.   wear a mask anytime they enter the room.

b.   wear a mask if they come within three feet of the client.

c.   not wear a mask if they have had tuberculosis.

d.   wait until the client has completed therapy to visit.

c
Comprehension
implementation
Safety: Safety and
Infection Control

30-30   Which of the following represents correct action following a potential exposure to bloodborne pathogens?

a.   Begin postexposure prophylaxis within 24 hours.

b.   Require the source individual to be tested for HIV/hepatitis.

c.   Test the exposed person for hepatitis immunity.

d.   Complete an injury report if the exposure requires treatment.

b
Application
Diagnosis
Psychosocial: coping
and adaptation

30-31   A male client is diagnosed with mononucleosis and does not want anyone know he has this disease. Which nursing diagnosis is appropriate for this client?

a.   Altered Thought Process: harmful feelings related to having an infectious disease

b.   Situation Low Self-Esteem related to negative feelings about having this disease

c.   Diversional Activity Deficit related to boredom from staying in the house.

d.   Fear related to negative thoughts that friends would not like him anymore.

c
Application
Planning
Physiological:
Physiological
Adaptation

30-32   A client with an infection has a nursing diagnosis of Alteration in Nutrition: Less than Body Requirements related to painful swallowing and anorexia. Select the appropriate nursing action.

a.   Total intake and output every four hours.

b.   Provide complex carbohydrates to eat.

c.   Offer soothing high protein liquids to drink.

d.   Provide warm liquids every two hours.

30-33 A nurse used her forceps to pack a purulent wound. After disposing of the old dressings, which intervention should she perform next?

    a. Rinse the forceps in cold water.

    b. Wash the forceps in hot, soapy water.

    c. Use a scrub brush to remove any foreign matter.

    d. Rinse the forceps in very hot water.

30-34 The nurse demonstrates correct practice of surgical asepsis when he:

    a. considers only objects above arm-level to be sterile.

    b. treats any item of uncertain sterility as contaminated.

    c. considers the surgeon's judgment of breach of technique to be the most accurate.

    d. holds the hands below the elbows during surgical handwashing and scrubbing.

30-35 In teaching home care to a client with an infection, which intervention would provide sterilization of the cotton mesh dressings?

    a. Steam the dressings 15 minutes.

    b. Hang the dressings out in the sun for 30 minutes.

    c. Boil the dressings for 20 minutes.

    d. Heat the dressings in a 400-degree oven for 10 minutes.

30-36 Which statement by the mother of a newborn indicates understanding of teaching to prevent infections?

    a. "The baby can use the same towel as my 2-year old."

    b. "The bottle can stay in the baby's room until the next feeding."

    c. "It would be better to keep my fingernails short and clean."

    d. "It is okay to wash the baby's clothes and diapers together."

<table>
<tr><td>

b
Application
Analysis/Diagnosis
Safety: Safety and
Infection Control

</td><td>

31-1   Which client is at risk for injury because of diminished ability to protect himself?

    a.   one who did not finish high school

    b.   one who is deaf

    c.   one who works in a law firm

    d.   one who is bored with his marriage

</td></tr>
</table>

b
Application
Analysis/Diagnosis
Safety: Safety and
Infection Control

31-1 Which client is at risk for injury because of diminished ability to protect himself?

a. one who did not finish high school

b. one who is deaf

c. one who works in a law firm

d. one who is bored with his marriage

c
Comprehension
Analysis/Diagnosis
Safety: Safety and
Infection Control

31-2 Which hospitalized client is at highest risk for injury?

a. a client with a newly diagnosed tumor

b. a teenager with many visitors

c. a recently admitted client in alcohol withdrawal

d. a postpartum mother who delivered two hours ago

d
Knowledge
Assessment
Safety: Safety and
Infection Control

31-3 What should a hazard appraisal of an adult's home include?

a. the number of bedrooms and bathrooms

b. the appraised value of the house

c. the age of the house

d. the adequacy of lighting in bedrooms and halls

b
Application
Analysis/Diagnosis
Physiological:
Reduction of Risk
Potential

31-4 A 75-year-old client has been hospitalized because of a stroke. He has left-sided weakness but is permitted to ambulate with a walker. An appropriate safety-related nursing diagnosis for this client is:

a. Activity Intolerance related to stroke.

b. Risk for Trauma related to left-sided weakness.

c. Powerlessness related to paralysis.

d. Risk for Aspiration related to stroke.

d
Comprehension
Implementation
Safety: Safety and
Infection Control

31-5 A 75-year-old client has been hospitalized because of a stroke. He has left-sided weakness but is permitted to ambulate with a walker. To promote the client's safety, the nurse should:

a. keep him on strict bedrest.

b. keep one of the bed side rails down at night.

c. apply a bed jacket restraint.

d. explain how to use the call bell system.

31-6   A 75-year-old client has been hospitalized because of a stroke. He has left-sided weakness but is permitted to ambulate with a walker. Because the client is older, what other factor besides weakness might increase his risk for physical injury?

a.   decreased ability to learn

b.   inability to reason

c.   altered nutritional status

d.   decreased sensory acuity

31-7   A 75-year-old client has been hospitalized because of a stroke. He has left-sided weakness but is permitted to ambulate with a walker. To ensure the client's safety when he is out of bed, the nurse should:

a.   restrict his activity to use of a wheelchair.

b.   follow him with a wheelchair as he walks.

c.   see that he wears nonskid footwear.

d.   apply a Posey restraint when he is in the chair.

31-8   Which fire extinguisher is appropriate to use on a paper or wood fire?

a.   water pump

b.   special dry powder

c.   dry chemical

d.   carbon dioxide

31-9   Which fire extinguisher is appropriate to use on both grease and electrical fires?

a.   water pump

b.   foam

c.   carbon dioxide

d.   special dry powder

31-10   A nurse who discovers a fire should first:

a.   use an extinguisher to put out the fire.

b.   notify the switchboard so an alarm can be sounded.

c.   evacuate clients in immediate danger.

d.   break the glass to activate a fire alarm.

d Knowledge Implementation Physiological: Pharmacological and Parenteral Therapies	31-11	In which situation would restraints be most useful? a. when the nurse is too busy to frequently check on an elderly client b. when trying to prevent a client from falling or other injury c. when trying to teach a client not to get up and go to the bathroom without assistance d. when movement of the client's arm would disrupt intravenous therapy
c Knowledge Planning Safety: Safety and Infection Control	31-12	Which type of restraint would allow the most movement by a client? a. jacket restraint b. wrist restraint c. mitt restraint d. mummy restraint
b Application Planning Safety: Safety and Infection Control	31-13	A seven-year-old client is admitted to the pediatric unit with eczema and keeps trying to scratch the skin lesions. The most effective type of restraint the nurse could use is a(n): a. wrist restraint. b. elbow restraint. c. jacket restraint. d. mummy restraint.
a Knowledge Implementation Physiological: Reduction of Risk Potential	31-14	A seven-year-old client has been restrained to keep her from scratching her skin lesions. How often should the nurse assess the restraints? a. every 30 minutes b. every 1 hour c. every 4 hours d. once a shift
a Knowledge Planning Safety: Safety and Infection Control	31-15	A nurse is teaching a preschool child about safety. Which age-specific hazards should the nurse emphasize? a. traffic injuries b. sports injuries c. substance abuse d. firearms
c Knowledge Planning Safety: Safety and Infection Control	31-16	Adolescent poisonings are most likely to be caused by which factor? a. inadequate supervision b. improper storage of toxic household substances c. recreational drugs or d. an overdose of a prescribed medication

d
Knowledge
Planning
Safety: Safety and
Infection Control

31-17 When teaching parents to prevent poisoning, the nurse should advise them:

    a. to reuse empty milk cartons to store lawn and garden chemicals.

    b. to administer syrup of ipecac whenever it is suspected that a child has ingested a poisonous substance.

    c. to say that medicine is candy so that children will take it more readily.

    d. not to take medications with great enjoyment in front of children.

b
Knowledge
implementation
Safety: Safety and
Infection Control

31-18 Which factor reduces the risk of electrical hazards?

    a. two-pronged electrical plugs

    b. three-pronged electrical plugs

    c. noninsulated wiring in the home

    d. using frayed cords cautiously

c
Knowledge
Implementation
Physiological:
Reduction of Risk
Potential

31-19 When caring for a client with radioactive implants the nurse should:

    a. wear shoes with rubber soles.

    b. use a mask when in close contact with the client.

    c. wear a lead apron when in close contact with the client.

    d. wear eye protection.

a
Comprehension
Implementation
Safety: Safety and
Infection Control

31-20 Which activity is correct when using a bed/chair exit safety monitoring device?

    a. The nurse applies the leg band to fit securely.

    b. The nurse plugs the device into a three-hole electrical outlet.

    c. The nurse fastens the device around the client's waist.

    d. The nurse lowers the side rails of the bed before leaving the room.

b
Application
Planning
Safety: Safety and
Infection Control

31-21 The nurse is planning to teach accident prevention to a 70-year-old client who lives alone. Which point would the nurse want to emphasize in the teaching plan?

    a. A throw rug at the foot of the stairs can cushion a fall.

    b. Keep a flashlight by the bed with good batteries.

    c. Keep all doors locked day and night.

    d. Do not give credit card information to solicitors.

c
Application
Diagnosis
Promotion: Growth
and Development
Through the Life
Span

31-22 Which NANDA nursing diagnosis is specific to school-aged children?

    a. Risk for Poisoning

    b. Risk for Suffocation

    c. Risk for Trauma

    d. Risk for Aspiration

31-23 Which statement by the parents of an infant indicates they understand safety measures for their baby?

   a. "A crib with wide spaces between the slats is safest."

   b. "I can prop the baby's bottle when I am busy with the two-year-old."

   c. "The car seat can fit in the front passenger seat."

   d. "Large soft toys without little parts are best right now."

31-24 The home health nurse noted many small burns in the client's sheets. He writes the nursing diagnosis Risk for Suffocation related to lack of home safety precautions. Which goal statement is most appropriate?

   a. Client will reduce the risk of suffocation as evidenced by absence of burns on sheets at next home visit.

   b. Client will state two home safety precautions by next week's visit.

   c. Client will not experience problems from lack of safety precautions during the week.

   d. Client will express feelings about home health and safety by the nurse's return visit.

31-25 A nursing diagnosis of Risk for Injury related to vertigo secondary to orthostatic hypotension is written for a client who complains of dizziness when getting out of bed. Which intervention should the nurse perform first?

   a. Have client wear slippers when getting up.

   b. Stand client at the bedside for a few moments before walking.

   c. Assist the client to rise slowly from a lying to a sitting position.

   d. Raise the bed to a comfortable height for the nurse.

d
Comprehension
Analysis/Diagnosis
Promotion: Growth
and Development
Through the Life
Span

32-1   When helping an elderly client bathe, the nurse also assesses his skin. Which finding is unexpected?

     a.   When pinched, the skin returns to place quickly.

     b.   The skin of the face, arms, and legs is intact.

     c.   The skin on the client's arms is smooth with some hair.

     d.   The client has several abrasions on his chest and back.

d
Comprehension
Analysis/Diagnosis
Physiological:
Physiological
Adaptation

32-2   Which client is at risk for developing impaired skin integrity?

     a.   one who is well hydrated

     b.   one who has an unpleasant body odor

     c.   one who is continent of urine and feces

     d.   one who has diminished sensation in the extremities

a
Knowledge
Implementation
Physiological: Basic
Care and Comfort

32-3   For a client confined to bed, which nursing activity is a part of the routine 'hour of sleep' care but not for 'early morning' care?

     a.   providing a back massage

     b.   providing a bedpan or urinal

     c.   changing the linen

     d.   washing the face and hands

b
Application
Planning
Physiological: Basic
Care and Comfort

32-4   "Moisture in contact with the skin for a period of time can result in increased bacterial growth and irritation." Which nursing intervention reduces the risk?

     a.   application of lanolin creams

     b.   application of non-irritating dusting powder

     c.   keeping bottom bed sheets taut and wrinkle free

     d.   use of bed cradle and footboard

c
Application
Planning
Physiological: Basic
Care and Comfort

32-5   A female client has an unpleasant body odor. What should the nurse do?

     a.   Apply non-irritating dusting powder to the client's axillae and perineum.

     b.   Shave the axillae and immediately apply underarm deodorant.

     c.   Make sure that the client's skin is clean, and apply underarm deodorant.

     d.   Apply lanolin lotion to her buttocks and perineum.

32-6 An assessment of the client's feet reveals a hard, flat, thickened portion of epidermis on both heels and the sides of both great toes. The client states that these areas are painless. The nurse recognizes these as:

a. calluses.

b. corns.

c. plantar warts.

d. bunions.

32-7 For a client with tinea pedis, which nursing order would be appropriate?

a. Apply antiseptic to gauze, insert between affected toes, and leave in place.

b. Dry feet well after bathing and allow to air dry. Apply clean stockings daily.

c. Soak feet in warm water with epsom salts, then abrade with pumice stone.

d. Apply salicylic acid followed by foot powder.

32-8 Which client needs special caution when you are providing foot care? One who:

a. one who is on bedrest

b. one who has diabetes

c. one who is confused

d. one who is ambulatory

32-9 The nurse is preparing to give oral care to an unconscious client. How should the nurse proceed?

a. Put the bed in high Fowler's position before beginning.

b. Lower the head of the bed, and place the client in side-lying position.

c. Put the client in Fowler's position, then turn her head to the side.

d. Place the client supine with her head lowered.

32-10 Which type of contact lens would cause the most serious concern if discovered in the eyes of an unconscious, nonblinking client?

a. hard

b. soft

c. gas permeable

d. disposable

32-11   Which intervention is a part of the correct procedure to follow in caring for a client's ears?

a.   If unable to loosen cerumen by retracting auricle, irrigate the canal.

b.   Retract the auricle upward to loosen visible cerumen.

c.   Use a syringe to aspirate cerumen from the ear canal.

d.   Have the client gently remove cerumen with a cotton-tipped applicator.

32-12   A client's hair should be combed and brushed:

a.   daily.

b.   twice daily.

c.   only when washed.

d.   weekly.

32-13   A male client scratches his head constantly. When examining his hair and scalp, the nurse notices small, oval, dandruff-like particles clinging to his hair, as well as small reddened lesions on his hair line. The nurse recognizes these as symptoms of:

a.   Lyme disease.

b.   pediculosis capitis.

c.   scabies.

d.   hirsutism.

32-14   It has just been discovered that a client has scabies. Which item would provide evidence that treatment and nursing care have been effective?

a.   The client verbalizes relief from nausea.

b.   The client does not develop Lyme disease.

c.   No further hair loss occurs.

d.   The parasites are not spread to other people.

32-15   When analyzing data regarding an elderly client's hair, the nurse should recognize that the hair of elderly clients normally:

a.   grows very fast.

b.   is very thick.

c.   tends to be oily.

d.   loses its color.

32-16 When providing perineal care for a female client, the correct procedure is to wipe:

 a. the area in concentric circular motions around the rectum.

 b. from the rectum toward the pubis.

 c. from the pubis toward the rectum.

 d. in concentric circles around the vaginal area.

32-17 A device used in hospitals to decrease pressure of the top bed covers on the client's feet, legs, and abdomen is a:

 a. bed cradle (Anderson frame).

 b. footboard.

 c. CircOlectric bed.

 d. Stryker frame.

32-18 Which action demonstrates correct bedmaking procedure?

 a. The nurse shakes crumbs from the soiled linen before placing it in the hamper.

 b. The nurse places the clean linen pack on the bedside table of client in bed A while making the bed of the client in bed B.

 c. The nurse wears sterile gloves while changing a client's bed linen.

 d. The nurse is careful not to bring soiled linens in contact with his uniform.

32-19 In making a hospital bed, which action describes correct application of sheets?

 a. The hem edge on the bottom sheet faces down and on the top sheet faces down.

 b. The hem edge on the bottom sheet faces down and on the top sheet faces up.

 c. The hem edge on the bottom sheet faces up and on the top sheet faces up.

 d. The hem edge on the bottom sheet faces up and on the top sheet faces down.

32-20 After cleaning and reinserting a hearing aid, the client reports a whistling sound. The nurse should:

 a. turn the volume down.

 b. turn the volume up.

 c. turn the hearing aid off.

 d. change the battery.

c
Application
Analysis/Diagnosis
Physiological:
Physiological
Adaptation

32-21   The nurse gathers the following data for a client who is unconscious: coated tongue, dry mouth, unpleasant breath odor, reddened gums. These are defining characteristics of:

    a.   Self-Care Deficit: (Oral) Hygiene.

    b.   Knowledge Deficit (Correct Oral Hygiene Practices).

    c.   Altered Oral Mucous Membrane.

    d.   Altered Nutrition: Less than Body Requirements.

d
Comprehension
Planning
Physiological: Basic
Care and Comfort

32-22   Which information is correct to teach a client about care of the teeth?

    a.   Floss the teeth daily.

    b.   Have an annual checkup by a dentist.

    c.   Begin taking your child to the dentist when he or she starts school.

    d.   Brush the teeth thoroughly after meals and at bedtime.

d
Comprehension
Implementation
Physiological: Basic
Care and Comfort

32-23   Which action demonstrates correct technique for eye care for the comatose client?

    a.   The nurse cleans the eyes with glucose solution and cotton balls.

    b.   The nurse instills mineral oil into the lower lids to lubricate the conjunctiva.

    c.   If the corneal reflex is absent, the nurse tapes saline soaked pads tightly over the eyes to keep the eyes closed.

    d.   The nurse cleans the eyes with saline solution, wiping from the inner canthus to the outer canthus.

a
Application
Evaluation
Promotion:
Prevention and Early
Detection of Disease

32-24   The home health nurse wants to evaluate the mother's understanding of measures to prevent tooth decay in her children. Which statement indicates the mother understands the teaching?

    a.   "Their teeth need to be flossed daily."

    b.   "Even young children can brush their teeth properly."

    c.   "Sweet foods are less harmful if eaten between meals."

    d.   "I should have a dentist check their teeth once a year."

c
Application
Implementation
Physiological: Basic
Care and Comfort

32-25   To shave a client with a safety razor, the nurse should first:

    a.   apply shaving cream to the face.

    b.   pat lotion on the skin .

    c.   put on clean gloves.

    d.   shave in short, firm strokes.

c
Application
Implementation
Physiological: Basic
Care and Comfort

32-26 An 80-year-old client had hip surgery yesterday. She is disoriented and has arthritis in her hands. Which type of bath should the nurse choose for this client?

a. tub bath

b. partial bath

c. complete bed bath

d. therapeutic bath

b
Application
Evaluation
Physiological: Basic
Care and Comfort

32-27 Which statement indicates the client understands the teaching regarding proper nail care?

a. "It is best to cut the nails one-half inch longer than the end of the fingers.

b. "I should use lotion to lubricate the skin around my nails."

c. "First, I need to cut my nails to fit the contour of my fingers."

d. "After biting my nails, I should use antibiotic ointment to prevent infection."

b
Knowledge
Implementation
Physiological:
Pharmacological and
Parenteral Therapies

33-1 Some medications are in the form of a powdered drug compressed into a small, hard disc. These medications can sometimes be broken on a scored line; others are enteric-coated. This type of drug preparation is a:

    a. pill.

    b. tablet.

    c. capsule.

    d. lozenge.

c
Knowledge
Implementation
Physiological:
Pharmacological and
Parenteral Therapies

33-2 The amount of time required for the body's elimination process to reduce the concentration of a drug to one-half what it was at initial administration is called the:

    a. onset of action.

    b. peak plasma level.

    c. drug half-life.

    d. plateau.

c
Knowledge
Implementation
Physiological:
Pharmacological and
Parenteral Therapies

33-3 The name given to a drug by the drug manufacturer is referred to as its:

    a. generic name.

    b. chemical name.

    c. brand name.

    d. official name.

c
Knowledge
Implementation
Physiological:
Pharmacological and
Parenteral Therapies

33-4 What does the Controlled Substance Act do?

    a. Prevent drug abuse and dependency.

    b. Provide treatment and rehabilitation for drug users.

    c. Categorize controlled substances.

    d. Identify drugs that can be sold only by prescription.

b
Knowledge
Assessment
Physiological:
Pharmacological and
Parenteral Therapies

33-5 A secondary, or unintended, effect of a drug on the body is called a:

    a. cumulative effect.

    b. side effect.

    c. toxic effect.

    d. drug interaction.

a
Knowledge
Assessment
Physiological:
Pharmacological and
Parenteral Therapies

33-6 Societally defined inappropriate intake of a substance, either continually or periodically, is called drug:

a. abuse.

b. misuse.

c. noncompliance.

d. addiction.

a
Knowledge
Implementation
Physiological:
Pharmacological and
Parenteral Therapies

33-7 A sweetened and aromatic solution of alcohol used as a vehicle for medicinal agents is a(n):

a. elixir.

b. extract.

c. spirit.

d. syrup.

c
Knowledge
Implementation
Physiological:
Pharmacological and
Parenteral Therapies

33-8 The administration of a medication under the tongue is called:

a. buccal.

b. oral.

c. sublingual.

d. lacrimal.

c
Knowledge
Implementation
Physiological:
Pharmacological and
Parenteral Therapies

33-9 The administration of a medication just under the skin is called:

a. intramuscular.

b. intradermal.

c. subcutaneous.

d. intravenous.

c
Knowledge
Implementation
Physiological:
Pharmacological and
Parenteral Therapies

33-10 When local medication is applied to the skin or the mucous membranes, the nurse charts that it has been given:

a. subcutaneously.

b. parenterally.

c. topically.

d. by inhalation.

b
Knowledge
Implementation
Physiological:
Pharmacological and
Parenteral Therapies

33-11 When a medication is injected into the body with a needle and syringe, it is administered:

a. intravenously.

b. parenterally.

c. topically.

d. intramuscularly.

a
Knowledge
Implementation
Physiological:
Pharmacological and
Parenteral Therapies

33-12   A knob on the upper femur which is used to help locate the dorsogluteal and ventrogluteal injection sites is the:

a. greater trochanter.

b. posterior iliac spine.

c. anterior superior iliac spine.

d. acromion process.

c
Comprehension
Implementation
Physiological:
Pharmacological and
Parenteral Therapies

33-13   A nurse is to give a client a medication for pain. The order is for morphine 40 mg. The PDR states the normal dose is 10 mg. The nurse should:

a. administer the ordered amount.

b. administer the normal dose.

c. contact the physician concerning the written order.

d. ask the head nurse if it safe to give the ordered amount.

c
Application
Implementation
Physiological:
Pharmacological and
Parenteral Therapies

33-14   The order reads, "Give morphine 10 mg. IM x1 at 0800." This is called a:

a. stat order.

b. prn order.

c. single order.

d. standing order.

a
Application
Implementation
Physiological:
Pharmacological and
Parenteral Therapies

33-15   Which of the following medication orders contains all of the essential parts needed for accurate drug administration?

a. 1-6-04, client's name, Demerol 100 mg, IM, q4h, prn pain, physician's signature

b. 1-5-04, morphine sulfate gr 1/6 stat, physician's signature

c. 1-1-04, client's name, Imferon, 1 cc, qod, physician's signature

d. 1-4-04, client's name, Lanoxin 0.125 mg, po, physician's signature

c
Knowledge
Implementation
Physiological:
Pharmacological and
Parenteral Therapies

33-16   Which medication order will be given most often?

a. bid

b. tid

c. qid

d. qod

c
Knowledge
Assessment
Physiological:
Pharmacological and
Parenteral Therapies

33-17   When completing a medication history, what should the nurse ask the client?

a. "Do you get up during the night to use the bathroom?"

b. "Do you exercise regularly?"

c. "Are you allergic to anything?"

d. "Has your appetite changed lately?"

d
Application
Implementation
Physiological:
Pharmacological and
Parenteral Therapies

33-18   The client is in the bathroom. When the nurse enters the room to give her medications, the client asks her to leave the pills on the bedside table. What should the nurse do?

a.   Leave the medication on the bedside table.

b.   Wait in the room until the client comes out of the bathroom.

c.   Go into the bathroom and give the client her pills.

d.   Tell the client she will return in a little while with the pills.

a
Application
Implementation
Physiological:
Pharmacological and
Parenteral Therapies

33-19   The primary nurse has prepared a preoperative IM injection for client A. Suddenly, client B becomes entangled in IV tubing and yells for help. The primary nurse rushes to assist client B. The surgery orderly is waiting for client A to have her preoperative medication, so the primary nurse asks another RN to give the injection to client A so she can go to surgery. What should the other RN do?

a.   Help client B so the primary nurse can give the preoperative injection.

b.   Give client A her preoperative medication.

c.   Prepare a new syringe for client A.

d.   Explain to the primary nurse that she cannot give the injection for him.

d
Comprehension
Implementation
Physiological:
Pharmacological and
Parenteral Therapies

33-20   The nurse is to give a three-year-old child an oral liquid medication. To facilitate the process, the nurse should:

a.   ask the child if she is ready to take the medication now.

b.   mix the medication with milk to disguise the taste.

c.   restrain the child while another nurse gives the medication.

d.   allow the child to choose whether to take the medication from a spoon or a plastic syringe.

c
Application
Implementation
Physiological:
Pharmacological and
Parenteral Therapies

33-21   The physician has ordered Demerol 35 mg, IM, q3h prn pain to be given to a client. The prefilled syringe of Demerol you have available reads 'Demerol 50 mg per ml'. You would administer to the client:

a.   0.35 ml.

b.   0.5 ml.

c.   0.7 ml.

d.   1.0 ml.

b
Application
Implementation
Physiological:
Pharmacological and
Parenteral Therapies

33-22   The physician orders penicillin 50,000 units for a client. You have available a 10 ml vial labeled '100,000 units per cc'. How much will you give?

a.   0.05 cc

b.   0.5 cc

c.   1.0 cc

d.   2.0 cc

33-23   Which physiologic change influences the administration of medications to elderly clients?

a.   There is an increase in renal blood flow, resulting in rapid uptake of medications from the bloodstream.

b.   There is less complete and slower absorption from the gastrointestinal tract, causing delayed onset after administration.

c.   There is increased proportion of lean body mass to fat, which increases the potential for toxicity of fat-soluble drugs.

d.   There is faster biotransformation of drugs in the liver, and therefore, higher potency.

33-24   A nurse is to give a combination of Demerol 50 mg and Vistaril 50 mg IM to a client. The Demerol is available in an ampule labeled '100 mg/ml' and the Vistaril is available in a multiple dose vial labeled '50 mg/ml'. What is the total volume to be administered in the syringe?

a.   1 ml

b.   1.5 ml

c.   2 ml

d.   2.5 ml

33-25   A nurse is to give a combination of Demerol 50 mg and Vistaril 50 mg IM to a client. The Demerol is available in an ampule labeled '100 mg/ml', and the Vistaril is available in a multiple dose vial labeled '50 mg/ml'. In order to mix the two medications in one syringe, the nurse should first:

a.   inject air into the ampule and then into the vial.

b.   inject air into the vial and then into the ampule.

c.   withdraw the medication from the vial and then from the ampule.

d.   withdraw the medication from the ampule and then from the vial.

33-26   A client is 5'6" tall and weighs 160 pounds. The nurse has selected the gluteus medius muscle for an IM injection. Which size needle should be used?

a.   22 gauge, 1 to 1.5 inch

b.   25 gauge, 1 inch

c.   20 gauge, 3 inch

d.   25 gauge, 5/8 inch

c
Comprehension
Planning
Physiological:
Pharmacological and
Parenteral Therapies

33-27 The nurse is going to use the Z-track method to inject a medication. His rationale for doing this is that:

a. the client has sufficient muscle for this type of injection.

b. it is the only method to use when giving an injection in the gluteus medius muscle.

c. the medication is highly irritating to subcutaneous and skin tissues.

d. it is the safest and least painful way to give an injection.

c
Knowledge
Implementation
Physiological:
Pharmacological and
Parenteral Therapies

33-28 Which abbreviation means 'before meals'?

a. OD

b. ad lib

c. ac

d. pc

c
Comprehension
Evaluation
Physiological:
Pharmacological and
Parenteral Therapies

33-29 After giving a medication that frequently causes allergic responses, two symptoms the nurse should observe for is:

a. confusion and disorientation.

b. tachycardia and irregular heart rhythm.

c. skin rash and nausea.

d. headache and constipation.

d
Comprehension
Evaluation
Physiological:
Pharmacological and
Parenteral Therapies

33-30 The onset of a drug would be expected to occur most quickly after administration by which route?

a. oral

b. subcutaneous

c. intramuscular

d. intravenous

b
Application
Implementation
Physiological:
Pharmacological and
Parenteral Therapies

33-31 The nurse enters a client's room to administer two tablets of aspirin. The client states she is unable to swallow pills. The nurse should respond:

a. "It is pretty easy to swallow aspirin. Please give it a try."

b. "They will taste tart but it is okay to chew them up."

c. "I will need to call the physician about this."

d. "Let me see if I can give you a suppository instead."

c
Application
Evaluation
Physiological:
Pharmacological and
Parenteral Therapies

33-32 Which statement indicates the client understands the teaching plan for taking insulin?

a. "I can give insulin in the same place every day."

b. "It is okay to use the same syringe that my sister uses."

c. "I should buy insulin syringes with 28 gauge needles."

d. "I should spread the skin tight before giving the injection."

b
Application
Implementation
Physiological:
Pharmacological and
Parenteral Therapies

33-33　The nurse is explaining a medication to a client when the client states, "Will this medicine affect my baby? I may be pregnant." How should the nurse reply?

a. "I do not think this medicine will affect your unborn baby."

b. "This may affect your baby. I will notify the physician."

c. "This medicine may have some very bad consequences for your baby."

d. "It is better to wait and see if you are pregnant before worrying about this medicine's effect on the baby."

d
Application
Implementation
Physiological:
Pharmacological and
Parenteral Therapies

33-34　Which action should the nurse perform when giving an antibiotic through the nasogastric tube?

a. Put the small tablets in the tube unaltered and flush with water.

b. Crush the tablet and dissolve it in cold water.

c. Check for tube placement after the medicine has been given.

d. Flush the tube with 30 mL of water after giving the medicine.

c
Application
Implementation
Physiological:
Pharmacological and
Parenteral Therapies

33-35　A nurse is preparing an insulin injection for a client who is 5'4" and weighs 102 pounds. Which technique is best for this client?

a. Pinch the skin and inject at a 90-degree angle.

b. Stretch skin taut and inject at a 90-degree angle.

c. Pinch the skin and inject at a 45-degree angle.

d. Stretch skin taut and inject at a 45-degree angle.

b
Comprehension
Analysis/Diagnosis
Physiological:
Physiological
Adaptation

34-1   The emaciated client is at high risk for developing which of the following skin integrity problems?

     a.   blisters

     b.   pressure sores

     c.   pustules

     d.   stasis dermatitis

a
Application
Analysis/Diagnosis
Physiological:
Physiological
Adaptation

34-2   A bedridden client is admitted to the hospital with a wound that itches and is draining a secretion irritating to the surrounding skin. During your initial assessment you see that the skin around the wound is red, swollen, and broken. Which of the following would be the most appropriate nursing diagnosis?

     a.   Impaired Skin Integrity related to wound drainage

     b.   Impaired Skin Integrity related to immobility

     c.   Risk for Impaired Skin Integrity related to pruritis

     d.   Risk for Impaired Skin Integrity related to redness

c
Comprehension
Physiological:
Reduction of Risk
Potential

34-3   What is one important reason to prevent pressure ulcers?

     a.   Once a pressure ulcer develops, it cannot be cured.

     b.   If a pressure ulcer develops, it can be spread to other parts of the body.

     c.   Pressure ulcers increase a client's cost of care.

     d.   Pressure ulcers cannot be prevented.

d
Application
Assessment
Physiological:
Physiological
Adaptation

34-4   Which of the following clients is at greatest risk for developing a pressure ulcer?

     a.   a 50-year-old man hospitalized for spinal surgery

     b.   a 60-year-old man in a nursing home for three months, but who can still ambulate with help

     c.   an 80-year-old woman hospitalized for a head injury

     d.   an 80-year-old woman who cannot turn herself in bed

b
Knowledge
Physiological:
Physiological
Adaptation

34-5   What is the approximate incidence of pressure sores in hospital settings?

     a.   1% to 2%

     b.   3% to 9%

     c.   10% to 20%

     d.   21% to 28%

a Knowledge Physiological: Physiological Adaptation	34-6	A client has an ischemic wound. This means that there has been: a. a deficient blood supply to the tissue. b. damage to the small blood vessels. c. compression of the tissue. d. a combination of friction and pressure.
b Comprehension Analysis/Diagnosis Physiological: Physiological Adaptation	34-7	When the nurse turns a client, she notices that the skin over his left hip bone is very white. By the time she finishes positioning him on his right side, the spot has turned bright red. This is called: a. ischemia. b. reactive hyperemia. c. a pressure ulcer. d. anoxia.
d Application Analysis/Diagnosis Physiological: Physiological Adaptation	34-8	When the nurse turns a client, she notices that the skin over his left hip bone is very white. By the time she finishes positioning him on his right side, the spot has turned bright red. The client had been on his left side for two hours before being turned. Therefore, the nurse should be concerned that tissue damage has occurred if the redness is still present at the end of: a. 1 minute. b. 5 minutes. c. 15 minutes. d. 45 minutes.
b Comprehension Analysis/Diagnosis Physiological: Physiological Adaptation	34-9	How do weakness and fatigue contribute to a client developing a pressure ulcer? a. The client does not feel discomfort in the pressure area and so he does not shift positions. b. Lack of energy hinders the client's ability to change positions. c. The client's level of consciousness, and therefore awareness, is reduced so the client is immobile. d. The medications given to minimize weakness and fatigue cause hypoproteinemia and resultant edema.
c Comprehension Analysis/Diagnosis Physiological: Physiological Adaptation	34-10	The nurse understands that a client with edema is predisposed to pressure ulcers because of: a. decreased body utilization of vitamin C. b. maceration of the skin. c. increased distance between the capillaries and the cells. d. increased amount of padding between the skin and the bones.

a
Comprehension
Planning
Physiological:
Physiological
Adaptation

34-11   In caring for a client with urinary incontinence, what is a factor that predisposes a client to pressure ulcers that the nurse should consider?

a. Moisture promotes skin maceration and causes the epidermis to erode easily.

b. Digestive enzymes in urine contribute to skin excoriation.

c. Urine kills the protective microorganisms on the client's skin, thereby making the person prone to infection.

d. Bacteria in the urine colonize on the skin, making the skin prone to infection.

c
Comprehension
Planning
Promotion: Growth
and Development
Through the Life
Span

34-12   The elderly are at high risk for impaired skin integrity because they have:

a. generalized thickening of the epidermis.

b. increased vascularity in the dermis.

c. decreased elasticity due to changes in the collagen fibers of the dermis.

d. increased skin turgor due to changes in the sebaceous glands.

a
Knowledge
Analysis/Diagnosis
Physiological:
Physiological
Adaptation

34-13   A client has a red spot over her sacrum. It does not blanch when the nurse presses on it. What stage of pressure ulcer formation does this represent?

a. Stage I

b. Stage II

c. Stage III

d. Stage IV

c
Knowledge
Analysis/Diagnosis
Physiological:
Physiological
Adaptation

34-14   A client has a pressure ulcer with necrosis of subcutaneous tissue. It looks like a deep crater, but it does not extend deeper than the subcutaneous tissue. What stage of pressure ulcer formation does this represent?

a. Stage I

b. Stage II

c. Stage III

d. Stage IV

a
Knowledge
assessment
Promotion:
Prevention and Early
Detection of Disease

34-15   When should the initial risk assessment for pressure ulcers be performed?

a. when the client is admitted to the institution

b. within 24 to 48 hours after the client is admitted to the institution

c. at least 24 hours after the client is admitted

d. before the client is discharged from the institution

34-16   When taking a culture from a wound, the nurse should obtain the sample from the:

    a.   edges of the wound.

    b.   area showing clean granulation.

    c.   deep section of the wound.

    d.   area with significant drainage.

34-17   A client has been lying on her back for two hours. When the nurse turns her, she notices that the skin over her sacrum is very white. By the time she finishes repositioning her, the spot has turned bright red. The nurse should:

    a.   massage the spot with lotion.

    b.   apply a warm compress for 30 minutes.

    c.   return in 30 to 45 minutes to see if the redness has disappeared.

    d.   wash the area with soap and water and notify the physician.

34-18   If the nurse determines that a client has a Stage I pressure ulcer, what would be the best desired outcome for a diagnosis of Impaired Skin Integrity?

    a.   The client will be able to reposition herself independently.

    b.   Skin will not become ulcerated.

    c.   Ulcer will not become infected.

    d.   The client will tolerate daily debridement.

34-19   To reduce shearing force for a bedridden client, it is most important for the nurse to:

    a.   put the bed in high Fowler's position.

    b.   pull the client up in bed at least once an hour.

    c.   wash the area daily with water and soap.

    d.   elevate the head of the bed no more than 30 degrees.

34-20   Using Norton's pressure area risk assessment form or the Braden scale for predicting pressure sore risk, which client is at highest risk for developing a pressure ulcer?

    a.   one with a score of 12

    b.   one with a score of 15

    c.   one with a score of 8

    d.   one with a score of 23

b
Knowledge
Implementation
Physiological:
Physiological
Adaptation

34-21 Which type of dressing should be used to debride necrotic tissue from a pressure ulcer?

a. impregnated nonadherent gauze

b. moist-to-dry gauze

c. transparent adhesive film

d. hydrocolloid

a
Application
Implementation
Physiological:
Reduction of Risk
Potential

34-22 Which nursing intervention should the nurse use for a client who is bedridden and has a nursing diagnosis of Impaired Skin Integrity related to prolonged bedrest?

a. Turn the client every 1.5 hours.

b. Change the client's position every 3 hours.

c. Use hot water to cleanse the client's skin.

d. Limit the client's fluids to 1500 mL/day.

b
Application
Evaluation
Physiological:
Reduction of Risk
Potential

34-23 Which statement by the client indicates an understanding of teaching regarding prevention of pressure ulcers?

a. "I should massage over bony areas to stimulate circulation."

b. "I need to change my position every 30 minutes."

c. "I will use a donut when I sit in the wheelchair."

d. "I will need to use baby oil to keep my skin lubricated."

b
Knowledge
Implementation
Physiological:
Reduction of Risk
Potential

34-24 Which of the following effects are produced by the initial application of heat?

a. vasoconstriction

b. increased capillary permeability

c. local anesthesia

d. slowed flow of pain impulses

c
Knowledge
Implementation
Physiological:
Reduction of Risk
Potential

34-25 What is the temperature range of tepid water?

a. 15 to 18° C (59 to 65° F)

b. 18 to 27° C (65 to 80° F)

c. 27 to 37° C (80 to 98° F)

c. 37 to 40° C (98 to 105° F)

a
Knowledge
Assessment
Physiological:
Physiological
Adaptation

34-26 An open wound resulting from friction is called a(n):

a. abrasion.

b. contusion.

c. incision.

d. laceration.

c
Comprehension
Assessment
Physiological:
Physiological
Adaptation

34-27   In assessing ecchymosis, it is important to note the:

    a. depth of the wound.

    b. condition of the wound edge.

    c. color and/or swelling.

    d. condition of the underlying tissue.

a
Comprehension
Assessment
Physiological:
Physiological
Adaptation

34-28   Which of the following is an example of a wound or injury that heals by secondary intention?

    a. burn

    b. fracture

    c. sprained ankle

    d. surgical incision

d
Knowledge
Planning
Physiological:
Physiological
Adaptation

34-29   Obesity compromises wound healing because:

    a. fatty tissue is fragile.

    b. there is more tissue to be healed.

    c. there is greater stress on the wound.

    d. fatty tissue usually has a limited blood supply.

b
Comprehension
Implementation
Physiological:
Reduction of Risk
Potential

34-30   In caring for a wound, the nurse cleans it by going from an area of least contamination to an area of greater contamination. The rationale for this technique is to:

    a. promote proper absorption of drainage.

    b. prevent contaminating previously cleaned areas.

    c. avoid reaching over cleaned areas.

    d. reduce excess moisture that may harbor microorganisms.

a
Application
Analysis/Diagnosis
Physiological:
Physiological
Adaptation

34-31   An adult client has just undergone an appendectomy. Two hours after returning from the recovery room, he requests medication for abdominal pain. His dressing is dry and intact. His vital signs are temperature 98.4° F, pulse 98, respirations 18, and BP 120/70. Based on this information alone, which of the following nursing diagnoses is most appropriate for him?

    a. Pain related to surgical procedure

    b. Inadequate Oxygenation related to pain

    c. Infection related to surgical incision

    d. Tachycardia related to blood loss

d
Comprehension
Assessment
Physiological:
Physiological
Adaptation

34-32 A client has just returned to his room after undergoing exploratory abdominal surgery. The nurse notes watery red drainage on his dressing. The nurse will describe the drainage as:

a. serous.

b. purulent.

c. sanguineous.

d. serous-sanguineous.

b
Application
Implementation
Physiological:
Physiological
Adaptation

34-33 When a client returns to his room after undergoing exploratory abdominal surgery, the nurse notes watery red drainage on his dressing. During the next four hours, the dressing becomes increasingly saturated with blood. The nurse should respond by:

a. calling the physician immediately.

b. adding more dressings and applying pressure.

c. applying a tourniquet around the closest artery.

d. removing the dressing and applying a fresh, dry dressing.

d
Knowledge
Assessment
Physiological:
Reduction of Risk
Potential

34-34 A 35-year-old client has been admitted for back surgery. She is 5'4" tall and weighs 120 pounds. She is divorced, a legal secretary, and the mother of two children. She has smoked one pack of cigarettes per day for the past 12 years. Which of the following factors in her history most adversely affects her wound healing?

a. weight

b. occupation

c. age

d. smoking

b
Application
Implementation
Physiological:
Reduction of Risk
Potential

34-35 Three days after abdominal surgery, a client rings for the nurse and says, "Something popped and gushed when I coughed." Several stitches are open and the incision edges are separate. The nurse should:

a. cover the area with dry, sterile abdominal pads.

b. cover the area with sterile towels soaked in sterile saline.

c. leave the area open to air.

d. apply an abdominal binder.

a
Application
Planning
Physiological:
Reduction of Risk
Potential

34-36 After a dehiscence, the physician orders frequent dressing changes. To prevent skin irritation from the frequent removal and replacement of the bandages, the nurses decide to use:

a. montgomery straps.

b. colloid spray.

c. large surgipads.

d. non-allergic gauze.

b
Comprehension
Planning
Physiological:
Reduction of Risk
Potential

34-37   The purpose of wet-to-damp dressings is to:

a.   occlude the wound.

b.   absorb exudate without disrupting new granulation tissue.

c.   heal the wound by primary intention.

d.   protect the wound from microorganisms.

c
Application
Implementation
Physiological:
Reduction of Risk
Potential

34-38   Which of the following techniques would be correct to use in applying a bandage to an extremity?

a.   Apply the bandage with the joint in extension to avoid strain.

b.   Work from the proximal to the distal end to promote blood flow.

c.   Leave the end of the limb exposed for circulation checks.

d.   Secure the bandage over the injured area to mark the exact location of the injury.

c
Knowledge
Analysis/Diagnosis
Physiological:
Reduction of Risk
Potential

34-39   A wound is considered infected if there is:

a.   redness.

b.   serous exudate.

c.   purulent exudate.

d.   eschar formation.

b
Knowledge
Analysis/Diagnosis
Physiological:
Reduction of Risk
Potential

34-40   After the maximum therapeutic effect of a thermal application has been achieved, the opposite effect begins. This is called the:

a.   adaptation response.

b.   rebound phenomenon.

c.   systemic effect.

d.   thermal reaction.

d
application
Planning
Physiological:
Reduction of Risk
Potential

34-41   For which client would heat therapy be contraindicated?

a.   a client with an edematous injury

b.   a client with impaired mobility

c.   a client who must go for an x-ray in an hour (so the heat will be applied for less than an hour)

d.   a client whose wound is still bleeding

c
Application
Implementation
Physiological:
Reduction of Risk
Potential

34-42   The nurse is applying a heating pad to a client's back. Which action is most appropriate?

a.   Remove the pad in one hour.

b.   Have the client lie on the pad.

c.   Use a pad with a preset heating switch.

d.   Pin the pad to the client's gown.

d
Application
Implementation
Physiological:
Physiological
Adaptation

34-43 The client's wound is located on the right wrist. Which method should the nurse use in securing the dressing?

a. Use montgomery straps for the wound.

b. Place strips of tape horizontally across the wrist.

c. Make sure the tape overlaps around the wrist.

d. Place the tape vertically across the wrist.

a
Application
Implementation
Physiological:
Physiological
Adaptation

34-44 A client has an open wound that is yellow and black. Using the RYB color code, which nursing intervention needs to occur first?

a. Debride the area with wet-to-dry dressings.

b. Apply topical antibiotic ointment.

c. Clean the wound gently.

d. Cover the wound with nonstick gauze.

a
Comprehension
Assessment
Physiological:
Physiological
Adaptation

35-1   What type of surgical procedure is a hip replacement?

    a.   transplant

    b.   palliative

    c.   diagnostic

    d.   constructive

d
Knowledge
Assessment
Physiological:
Reduction of Risk
Potential

35-2   A blood urea nitrogen or creatinine screening test is done routinely prior to surgery to assess the functioning of the:

    a.   lungs.

    b.   heart.

    c.   liver.

    d.   kidneys.

d
Knowledge
Assessment
Physiological:
Physiological
Adaptation

35-3   Which clinical sign would alert the nurse to possible postoperative hemorrhage?

    a.   elevated temperature

    b.   dyspnea

    c.   pain in incision

    d.   rapid, weak pulse

b
Knowledge
Planning
Physiological:
Reduction of Risk
Potential

35-4   The nurse ensures that the client is well hydrated in order to help prevent postoperative:

    a.   hemorrhage.

    b.   thrombophlebitis.

    c.   urinary retention.

    d.   wound infection.

a
Application
Evaluation
Physiological:
Reduction of Risk
Potential

35-5   Which of the following sets of client data would allow the nurse to conclude that the nursing actions taken to prevent postoperative pneumonia have been effective?

    a.   temperature 98.6° F, no cough, no dyspnea, no chest pain

    b.   pulse 80, respirations 20, skin color pink, skin warm and dry

    c.   intake = output, voiding normal amounts, no discomfort except in incision when moving in bed, temperature 98.6° F

    d.   no nausea or vomiting, appetite good, slept well last night

c Knowledge Physiological: Physiological Adaptation	35-6	Which perioperative phase begins when the client is transferred to the operating room table and ends when the client is transferred to the postanesthetic area? a. preoperative b. postoperative c. intraoperative d. transoperative
a Application Analysis/Diagnosis Physiological: Physiological Adaptation	35-7	Which client would be a logical candidate for a general anesthetic? a. a client who is extremely anxious about a surgery that cannot be postponed b. a client who is having a minor surgical procedure as an outpatient c. a client who has a serious chronic respiratory disease d. a client who has circulatory insufficiency
b Knowledge Planning Safety: Management of Care	35-8	Obtaining legal, informed consent to perform surgery is the responsibility of the: a. staff nurse. b. surgeon. c. nurse administrator. d. family physician.
d Knowledge Analysis/Diagnosis Physiological: Reduction of Risk Potential	35-9	Which of the following factors increases a client's risk of surgical complications? a. age 35 b. taking vitamins c. five pounds underweight d. dehydration
c Application Analysis/Diagnosis Psychosocial: Coping and Adaptation	35-10	During the admission interview, the client tells the nurse she is afraid she will not wake up after the surgery. A possible nursing diagnosis is: a. Anxiety related to perceived inability to deal with possible pain. b. Knowledge Deficit related to coping with postoperative pain. c. Fear related to unknown outcome of surgery. d. Ineffective Individual Coping related to surgery.
d Knowledge Analysis/Diagnosis Physiological: Reduction of Risk Potential	35-11	Which medication, if taken regularly, increases a client's surgical risk? a. vitamin C b. acetaminophen (Tylenol) c. thyroid replacement hormone d. anticoagulants

a	35-12	A male client has smoked 2 packs of cigarettes per day for the past 15

a
Comprehension
Analysis/Diagnosis
Physiological:
Reduction of Risk
Potential

35-12 A male client has smoked 2 packs of cigarettes per day for the past 15 years. This puts him at increased risk for developing:

    a. postoperative respiratory complications.

    b. intraoperative fluid and electrolyte imbalance.

    c. preoperative stress and anxiety.

    d. postoperative wound infection.

c
Comprehension
Planning
Psychosocial:
Coping and
Adaptation

35-13 What information should the nurse include in a client's preoperative teaching?

    a. a description of the different postoperative complications that must be prevented

    b. a detailed description of the surgical procedure to be performed

    c. postoperative plans for pain management

    d. explanation of the potential side effects of the anesthetic to be used

c
Application
Evaluation
Physiological:
Physiological
Adaptation

35-14 Which of the following outcomes would demonstrate the effectiveness of preoperative teaching?

    a. The client sleeps well the night before surgery.

    b. The client has a balanced intake and output.

    c. The client demonstrates deep breathing, coughing, splinting, and leg exercises.

    d. The client remains free of infection, as manifested by normal temperature.

b
Comprehension
Implementation
Psychosocial:
Coping and
Adaptation

35-15 A five-year-old client is to have a tonsillectomy. The nurse can best help allay the client's anxiety about surgery by:

    a. asking him what the doctors have told him about surgery.

    b. showing him the special clothes, rooms, and equipment that will be used.

    c. being open and honest and telling him exactly how many injections he will have.

    d. giving him a sedative.

c
Application
Implementation
Safety: Management
of Care

35-16 A nurse who speaks no Spanish must witness an operative permit signed by a client who speaks no English. The nurse should:

    a. have the physician get another witness.

    b. go ahead and witness the permit, since the physician is the one responsible for obtaining the consent.

    c. ask an interpreter to be present to help her to assess the client's understanding of the surgery and the permit.

    d. look through the chart to see if the client has any English-speaking relatives who might be able to come and witness the permit.

d
Application
Implementation
Physiological:
Physiological
Adaptation

35-17 A client is scheduled to undergo an exploratory laparotomy this morning. He has been NPO since midnight and is complaining that his mouth is very dry. The nurse should:

a. offer him a small sip of water or some ice chips.

b. give him a piece of hard candy to suck on.

c. explain that he cannot have anything in his mouth until after surgery.

d. encourage him to brush his teeth and rinse his mouth, but not to swallow the water.

a
Knowledge
Planning
Physiological:
Reduction of Risk
Potential

35-18 The purpose of antiembolism stockings is to:

a. facilitate the return of venous blood to the heart.

b. prevent varicose veins in the legs.

c. ensure joint mobility and prevent contractures.

d. prevent atrophy of the leg muscles.

a
Comprehension
Implementation
Physiological:
Reduction of Risk
Potential

35-19 To assure proper suctioning of a nasogastric tube, the nurse should:

a. check all the connections for leakage.

b. place the tubing below the suction bottle..

c. assure tube placement by injecting water into the tube and listening over the client's stomach.

d. assess the client once per shift.

c
Comprehension
Evaluation
Physiological:
Reduction of Risk
Potential

35-20 Placement of a nasogastric tube can be verified by:

a. shining a light on the client's oropharynx.

b. asking the client to swallow to see if the gag reflex is stimulated.

c. using a syringe to aspirate stomach contents and checking the acidity.

d. injecting 50 cc of water into the tube and listening over the stomach with a stethoscope.

c
Application
Analysis/Diagnosis
Physiological:
Physiological
Adaptation

35-21 A client has just undergone an appendectomy. Two hours after returning to the unit, he requests pain medication. His dressing is dry and intact. His vital signs are temperature 98.4° F, pulse 98, respirations 18, and BP 120/70. Based on this information, which nursing diagnosis is appropriate?

a. Pain related to surgical procedure

b. Body Image Disturbance related to extensive scarring

c. Infection related to surgical incision

d. Decreased Cardiac Output related to tachycardia

b
Comprehension
Assessment
Physiological:
Reduction of Risk
Potential

35-22 To most accurately assess tissue perfusion, the recovery room nurse should:

a. take vital signs.

b. check the color of the lips and nail beds.

c. assess respiratory movement.

d. monitor pedal pulses.

b
Application
Implementation
Physiological:
Reduction of Risk
Potential

35-23 A client has an incision with a penrose drain. What should the nurse do when he changes the dressing?

a. Remove the old dressing with a sterile glove.

b. Clean the incision site, then clean around the drain.

c. Use one swab to clean all around the drain and one inch below it.

d. Place most of the dressings above the drain site to absorb the drainage.

d
Comprehension
Implementation
Physiological:
Reduction of Risk
Potential

35-24 Which nursing intervention is appropriate during the first 24 hours after a client has had an abdominal surgery done under general anesthesia?

a. Remind the client not to try to turn from side to side, to prevent dehiscence.

b. Tell the client to ask for pain medication only if the pain becomes severe, as narcotics will further depress respirations.

c. If the client coughs during deep breathing exercises, notify the physician.

d. Give ice chips, if ordered, and mouthwash. Measure intake and output.

c
Application
Evaluation
Physiological:
Reduction of Risk
Potential

35-25 Which statement indicates the client's friend understands the home care instructions for wound care?

a. "If the wound is painful, I will give pain medication one hour before starting to change it."

b. "It is okay if his cat keeps him company while I change the dressing."

c. "I will report any increase in redness or swelling of the wound."

d. "It is okay to use adhesive tape since the skin is intact."

b
Application
Implementation
Physiological:
Reduction of Risk
Potential

35-26 A client with a chronic obstructive lung disease is scheduled for abdominal surgery. Which preoperative teaching is most important for this client?

a. Explain how to perform leg exercises.

b. Demonstrate coughing and deep breathing.

c. Encourage a large fluid intake postoperatively.

d. Apply antiembolism stockings.

35-27 Which nursing diagnosis has priority while the client is in the postanesthesia care unit?

a. Ineffective Airway Clearance related to the effects of anesthesia
b. Acute Pain related to discomfort when moving
c. Body Image Disturbance related to large abdominal incision
d. Knowledge Deficit related to lack of information about home care

b
Knowledge
Psychosocial:
Coping and
Adaptation

36-1   The conscious organization and translation of stimuli into meaningful information is called:

a. stereognosis.

b. sensory perception.

c. kinesthesia.

d. sensory reception.

c
Knowledge
Psychosocial:
Coping and
Adaptation

36-2   The ability to integrate environmental stimuli and body reactions and to respond accordingly is called:

a. sensorium.

b. cognition.

c. awareness.

d. kinesthesia.

d
Application
Assessment
Psychosocial:
Coping and
Adaptation

36-3   Which client would be at most risk of experiencing sensory disturbances?

a. a normal 8-week-old infant

b. a 24-year-old male in a lower leg cast

c. a 44-year-old female who left her reading glasses at home

d. a 56-year-old male in intensive care unit with myocardial infarction (heart attack)

a
Comprehension
Analysis/Diagnosis
Psychosocial:
Coping and
Adaptation

36-4   What is wrong with writing the nursing diagnosis Altered Thought Processes related to permanent physiologic changes secondary to aging?

a. A desired outcome would have to be the improvement of thought processes, and this is not possible for the nurse to achieve independently.

b. Altered thought processes are not usually related to physiologic changes.

c. The nurse can intervene independently to treat the problem, but not the etiology.

d. 'Altered Thought Processes' is not a NANDA diagnostic label.

b
Comprehension
Analysis/Diagnosis
Psychosocial:
Coping and
Adaptation

36-5   Which client is most at risk for sensory deficit?

a. a client who hallucinates frequently

b. a client with paralysis resulting from a spinal cord injury

c. a client who is being treated in the emergency room for a bleeding ulcer

d. a client who is waiting to be seen by a physician in a busy clinic

36-6 Hallucinations and delusions are two clinical problems that may appear with:

a. sensory deprivation.

b. sensory deficit.

c. sensory overload.

d. altered consciousness.

36-7 A 78-year-old client reports difficulty reading small print and driving, especially at night. She also reports she has difficulty getting up and down her stairs and that "they seem to blend together." Which nursing diagnosis is most appropriate for this client?

a. Sensory/Perceptual Alterations: Sensory Deprivation related to therapeutic isolation

b. Risk for Injury: Falls related to declining vision associated with aging

c. Sensory/Perceptual Alterations: Sensory Overload related to hospitalization

d. Altered Thought Processes related to hospitalization and aging

36-8 Which of the following nursing diagnoses is one for which the nurse can write independent nursing interventions?

a. Altered Thought Processes: Decreased Level of Consciousness related to head injury

b. Sensory/Perceptual Alterations: Visual related to eye surgery

c. Sensory/Perceptual Alterations: Auditory related to having had measles as a child

d. Risk for Injury: Falls related to sensory/perceptual alteration (impaired vision)

36-9 A client who is a quadriplegic has been placed on Clinitron flotation bed therapy for treatment of a decubitus ulcer. The noise of the motorized bed has been keeping him awake and he is becoming fatigued, agitated, and restless. The nurse's best intervention would be to:

a. inform the physician of the client's adverse reaction to the bed.

b. tell the client he must remain on the bed until his decubitus ulcer is healed, and encourage him to try to rest.

c. administer a tranquilizer during the day and sleeping medication at night to help him cope with the noxious sensory stimulus.

d. provide diversional activities during the day, and try to help the client reinterpret the motor hum as soothing and relaxing at night.

b
Application
Evaluation
Physiological:
Reduction of Risk
Potential

36-10 A client has a nursing diagnosis of Altered Sleep Patterns related to the noise from his motorized bed (a treatment for his decubitus ulcer). Which desired outcome most clearly indicates that his sensory disturbance is no longer a problem?

    a. Decubitus ulcer heals rapidly; granulation tissue appears within two weeks.

    b. Sleeps for six hours without awakening.

    c. Watches three television programs in succession during the day.

    d. Appears less fatigued and less restless.

c
Comprehension
Implementation
Physiological:
Physiological
Adaptation

36-11 A client has developed septicemia and lapsed into unconsciousness. His family stays with him around the clock. The nurse should encourage the family to:

    a. dim the lights and keep noise to a minimum.

    b. quietly and lightly touch and stroke the client.

    c. talk to and touch the client as if he was conscious.

    d. stay back from the bed so as not to disturb the client or be in the way.

c
Application
Planning
Physiological:
Reduction of Risk
Potential

36-12 A client has had a cerebral vascular accident and has lost visual acuity. When planning care, the nurse should provide:

    a. protective ear covers to prevent further hearing loss.

    b. a means by which the client can communicate her needs.

    c. a way to compensate for the client's loss of vision.

    d. active range-of-motion exercises for all extremities.

c
Comprehension
Implementation
Psychosocial:
Coping and
Adaptation

36-13 An 80-year-old widow recently became a resident of an extended care facility. Three days after she was admitted, the nurse found her to be somewhat confused and disoriented about person, place, and time. Which intervention by the nurse would be most appropriate?

    a. Use a posey restraint to keep the client from falling out of bed.

    b. Encourage diversional activities such as watching television.

    c. Reorient her to person, place, and time as often as possible.

    d. Touch and stroke her frequently.

d
Knowledge
Implementation
Psychosocial:
Coping and
Adaptation

36-14 Which intervention can improve communication with the hearing-impaired client?

    a. Use short phrases, which are easier to understand than longer ones.

    b. Frequently change the volume of your voice throughout each sentence.

    c. Talk at a slow rate and in a loud voice.

    d. Make sure the client can see your face easily and that the room is well lighted.

36-15   A client's nursing assessment includes the following data: client states that he feels alone and rejected by others; he has no family or friends in this city; he is withdrawn; he does not make eye contact. These defining characteristics suggest a NANDA nursing diagnosis of:

    a. Social Isolation.

    b. Altered Thought Processes.

    c. Impaired Home Maintenance Management.

    d. Sensory/Perceptual Alterations.

36-16   A client's vision is deteriorating. She says she is having difficulty preparing her meals. Which action might help to support her visual function?

    a. Suggest that she use colored rims on dishes and color-code dials on her stove.

    b. Suggest that she get her food from Meals on Wheels.

    c. Suggest that she have a home health aide come to prepare her meals.

    d. Suggest that she ask her husband to cook the meals.

36-17   Touching and stroking are specific nursing interventions for clients who are:

    a. aphasic.

    b. unconscious.

    c. disoriented.

    d. hearing impaired.

36-18   When planning meaningful stimulation for a client with sensory deprivation, it is most important that the nurse:

    a. provide a variety of stimuli so that the client will not be bored.

    b. include visual stimuli because that is the most important sense to most people.

    c. determine whether deprivation is due to inadequate stimuli or inability to receive or process stimuli.

    d. obtain a physician's order before stimulating the client.

36-19   The client's history indicates that she has smoked cigarettes for 25 years. Which sensory function should the nurse be especially sure to assess? Her sense of:

    a. smell.

    b. vision.

    c. hearing.

    d. touch.

c
Application
Planning
Psychosocial:
Coping and
Adaptation

36-20 The nurse wears a large name tag and introduces herself to the client each time she enters his room. She has placed a calendar and a clock in his room along with photographs of his family. These nursing interventions are specifically intended to:

a. support the client's hearing deficit.

b. support the client's visual deficit.

c. prevent sensory deprivation.

d. facilitate the client's stereognosis.

c
Application
Implementation
Physiological:
Reduction of Risk
Potential

36-21 Which safety measure should the nurse emphasize while teaching a client who has decreased tactile sensation in the lower extremities?

a. Maintain a constant temperature in the house.

b. Wear shoes with rubber soles when going outside.

c. Check temperature of bath water on the forearm before getting into tub.

d. Wear gloves and a hat when going out in cold weather.

b
Application
Evaluation
Physiological:
Reduction of Risk
Potential

36-22 The school nurse is teaching a class on health and safety to a group of second grade students. Which statement by one of the children indicates an understanding of safety measures to prevent sensory impairments?

a. "My mom takes me to see the nurse when I am sick."

b. "I wear goggles when my friend and I use a hammer."

c. "My baby sister grabbed a screwdriver off the table."

d. "My older brother plays his radio very, very loud."

a
Application
Evaluation
Safety: Safety and
Infection Control

36-23 Which statement by a client with decreased vision indicates safe adaptation to the home environment?

a. "I have had all the loose throw rugs taken up at my place."

b. "My dog and cat are not much trouble, and they keep me company."

c. "I know my family worries about me, but I don't want to leave my home."

d. "Since my eyes have weakened, my hearing is more acute."

c
Application
Assessment
Psychosocial:
Coping and
Adaptation

36-24 Which assessment data indicates the client has had an unexpected or detrimental change in sensory/perceptual functioning?

a. the client has worn contact lenses for the last five years

b. her partner states that the client does not like to eat cabbage

c. her partner states that the client does not answer telephone anymore

d. the client enjoys smelling fresh flowers in the house

b
Application
Evaluation
Psychosocial:
Coping and
Adaptation

36-25 A client in a nursing home has a nursing diagnosis of Social Isolation related to decreased visual acuity. Which outcome statement indicates the social isolation is resolving?

a. Wears glasses while in the room but not in the halls.
b. Joins a reading group that uses books with large print.
c. Has no injuries or skin tears for one month.
d. Eats at the assigned table in the dining room.

a
Application
Psychosocial:
Coping and
Adaptation

37-1   A registered nurse who is going back to college to obtain a baccalaureate degree in nursing is at times unsure what her actions should be in her clinical experiences. The staff nurses know she is an RN, so they have certain expectations of her, but her instructor expects her to complete her assignments as a student. This registered nurse is experiencing:

a.   role ambiguity.

b.   role strain.

c.   role performance.

d.   role mastery.

c
Knowledge
Assessment
Psychosocial:
Coping and
Adaptation

37-2   How an individual feels about himself/herself is referred to as:

a.   self-identity.

b.   body image.

c.   self-esteem.

d.   role performance.

a
Knowledge
Assessment
Psychosocial:
Coping and
Adaptation

37-3   The conscious sense of one's individuality and uniqueness is referred to as:

a.   self-identity.

b.   global self.

c.   body image.

d.   self-esteem.

b
Knowledge
Assessment
Psychosocial:
Coping and
Adaptation

37-4   The image of one's physical self is referred to as:

a.   self-identity.

b.   body image.

c.   personal self.

d.   self-esteem.

b
Knowledge
Analysis/Diagnosis
Psychosocial:
Coping and
Adaptation

37-5   The four components of self-concept as defined by the North American Nursing Diagnosis Association include body image, role performance, personal identity, and:

a.   self-image.

b.   self-esteem.

c.   global self.

d.   personal self.

37-6   When assessing a client's self-concept, the nurse should create a quiet environment, minimize interruptions, and:

   a.   sit at eye level with the client.

   b.   ask close-ended questions.

   c.   ask multiple personal questions.

   d.   confide in other family members.

37-7   While caring for a client, the nurse notices that her behavior indicates a negative resolution of the trust versus mistrust stage of psychosocial development. Which behavior is a likely cue to this inference by the nurse?

   a.   The client is overly concerned about being clean.

   b.   The client shares time, opinions, and experiences.

   c.   The client expresses curiosity about many things.

   d.   The client is unable to accept assistance.

37-8   Which behavior indicates that a client who is scheduled for surgery is positively resolving the integrity stage of psychosocial development?

   a.   He demands unnecessary assistance and attention from others.

   b.   He expresses his own opinion.

   c.   He accepts his own limitations.

   d.   He verbalizes anxiety about the surgery.

37-9   After a teaching session with the diabetes educator, the client tells the nurse, "I am too dumb and too old to do all this stuff." The nurse recognizes this to be a negative sense of:

   a.   self-concept and self-esteem.

   b.   behavior and self-perception.

   c.   global self.

   d.   social role fulfillment.

37-10   The client knows her pancreas is not functioning properly and that she is going to have to alter her eating habits and inject herself daily to provide the insulin her body needs for glucose metabolism. The nurse is aware that considerable anxiety may be created by this change in the client's:

   a.   role performance.

   b.   self-identity.

   c.   body image.

   d.   self-esteem.

a
Application
Analysis/Diagnosis
Psychosocial:
Coping and
Adaptation

37-11   The client tells the nurse that he is a retired railroad engineer and is considered an expert on air brake systems. This can be described as an expression of the client's:

a. sense of identity.

b. role ambiguity.

c. ego integrity.

d. self-ideal.

c
Comprehension
Assessment
Psychosocial:
Coping and
Adaptation

37-12   What is the most important influence on a person's ability to cope with a major stressor?

a. the specific nature of the stressor itself

b. the person's problem-solving abilities

c. the person's perception of the stressor

d. the availability of resources

c
Application
Analysis/Diagnosis
Psychosocial:
Coping and
Adaptation

37-13   The client has been in the hospital several weeks. She has stopped bathing and brushing her hair, and has been refusing to take telephone calls or see visitors. In response to the nurse's efforts at client teaching, she says, "I don't see why you bother. I won't be able to remember it anyway." What is the best nursing diagnosis for this client?

a. Risk for Impaired Coping

b. Altered Role Performance

c. Self-Esteem Disturbance

d. Body Image Disturbance

d
Application
Evaluation
Psychosocial:
Coping and
Adaptation

37-14   The client has been in the hospital several weeks. She has stopped bathing and brushing her hair, and has been refusing to take telephone calls or see visitors. One of the goals for her care is that she will perceive and respond to the stress of hospitalization in a constructive manner. The nurse can evaluate if that goal is being met when the client:

a. makes a new friend each day.

b. watches television and works crossword puzzles.

c. makes plans to adapt to a new role after dismissal.

d. participates in daily personal hygiene.

c
Comprehension
Assessment
Psychosocial:
Coping and
Adaptation

37-15   For a client with a nursing diagnosis of Self-Esteem Disturbance, the goal is that she will perceive and respond to the stress of hospitalization in a constructive manner. In order to develop interventions to meet this goal, it is most important for the nurse to assess the client's:

a. interests and past accomplishments.

b. involvement with significant others.

c. ideal and perceived self-concept.

d. intellectual and spiritual strengths.

c
Comprehension
Planning
Psychosocial:
Coping and
Adaptation

37-16 Which strategy would be most effective in enhancing the self-esteem of a school-age child?

a. Have as few rules as possible; for example, let the child set her own bedtime.

b. Communicate that there are no expectations for school achievement and that it is up to the child.

c. Set and consistently enforce well-defined limits to behavior.

d. Praise all efforts the child makes (for example, "Good job!").

a
Knowledge
Planning
Psychosocial:
Coping and
Adaptation

37-17 A nursing student is caring for two 4-year-old children. She remembers to give the children initiative to explore and act out various roles in their play, realizing that failure to achieve a sense of initiative can result in feelings of:

a. guilt.

b. mistrust.

c. shame and doubt.

d. role confusion.

c
Comprehension
Implementation
Psychosocial:
Coping and
Adaptation

37-18 How can the nurse enhance feelings of self-esteem and self-worth of an elderly client?

a. Determine the client's perceptions of physical self.

b. Plan the minutiae of the client's daily activities to remove the burden of decision making.

c. Ask permission before moving objects in the client's room.

d. Lay out the client's clothes so she will know what to put on each day.

c
Comprehension
Assessment
Psychosocial:
Coping and
Adaptation

37-19 The nurse is caring for a client with self-concept problems. To assess the specific stressors about role the nurse would assist the client to identify factors such as:

a. changes in physical appearance.

b. any type of disfigurement.

c. divorce or separation.

d. repeated failures.

b
Application
Implementation
Psychosocial:
Coping and
Adaptation

37-20 A client has a nursing diagnosis of Situational Low Self-Esteem related to starting nursing school and trying to maintain the home. Which strategy could the nurse use to assist this client?

a. Listen to negative thoughts from the client.

b. Encourage client to set realistic goals.

c. Gloss over slight imperfections.

d. Use humor by laughing at client's fears.

b
Application
Implementation
Psychosocial:
Coping and
Adaptation

37-21 A client had a mastectomy yesterday and refuses to look at the incision. A nursing diagnosis of Body Image Disturbance related to negative perceptions of her womanhood has been developed. The nurse could encourage her to identify personal strengths by:

a. insisting she look at the incision.
b. appealing to her sense of humor.
c. having her family look at the incision.
d. telling her there is always 'tomorrow'.

a
Application
Planning
Psychosocial:
Coping and
Adaptation

37-22 A client went to the clinic and had a nursing diagnosis of Situational Low Self-Esteem related to nursing school and trying to maintain the home. What is an appropriate goal?

a. Client will state two positive aspects of her life.
b. Client will hire help for the home.
c. Client will not be moody.
d. Client will stop school and take care of her family.

d
Application
Evaluation
Psychosocial:
Coping and
Adaptation

37-23 Which statement indicates the client has resolved negative feelings about low self-esteem?

a. "I'm not sure my friends will want to be around me."
b. "There is no way I can tackle this report now."
c. "Even though my friend is not kind to me, I will stick by him."
d. "Being successful one time means I can do it again."

c
Application
Evaluation
Psychosocial:
Coping and
Adaptation

37-24 Which statement indicates the client is resolving a negative image of his body following skin grafts for third-degree burns?

a. "I'm not sure my friends will want to be around me."
b. "I could be the freak at the circus now."
c. "With my hair combed to the side the graft is less noticeable."
d. "All the monster parts in the play will be easy for me to get now."

b Comprehension Implementation Promotion: Growth and Development Through the Life Span	**38-1** A 13-year-old student heard her friends talking about masturbation and asked her mother what they meant. Her mother's best explanation would be that masturbation is: a. physically unwholesome. b. a manual form of sexual self-stimulation. c. only done by the mentally ill. d. oral-genital stimulation by a sex partner.
d Knowledge Assessment Promotion: Growth and Development Through the Life Span	**38-2** Which finding is an indication that a woman is sexually excited? a. shrinking of her areola b. relaxation of her muscles c. decrease in her heart rate d. increase in her vaginal lubrication
d Comprehension Implementation Promotion: Growth and Development Through the Life Span	**38-3** A mother discovered her five-year-old son playing naked under the bed covers with another little boy. An understanding of and healthy reaction to this situation would be for her to: a. let him continue playing. b. restrict him to his room for the rest of the day. c. inform the other child's mother that her son is probably a homosexual. d. get the boys interested in another activity.
c Knowledge Planning Promotion: Growth and Development Through the Life Span	**38-4** A couple goes to see a counselor because they are having sexually related problems in their marriage. They ask the counselor what she would advise about having the husband orally stimulate his wife's genitals. This form of stimulation is called: a. anilingus. b. fellatio. c. cunnilingus. d. soixante-neuf.
c Knowledge Assessment Promotion: Growth and Development Through the Life Span	**38-5** The involuntary climax of sexual tension occurs during which phase of the sexual response cycle? a. excitement b. plateau c. orgasmic d. resolution

a
Application
Implementation
Promotion: Growth
and Development
Through the Life
Span

38-6   A couple goes to see a counselor because they are having sexually related problems in their marriage. The counselor advises that they might try to enhance their psychologic stimulation by:

    a. wearing perfume and cologne.

    b. leaving the television on during foreplay.

    c. wearing a condom.

    d. turning off the lights before attempting sexual intercourse.

b
Knowledge
Analysis/Diagnosis
Promotion: Growth
and Development
Through the Life
Span

38-7   A client was a victim of sexual incest as a child. Now, when she attempts to have intercourse, her vaginal muscles contract, preventing penile penetration. This condition is called:

    a. impotence.

    b. vaginismus.

    c. dyspareunia.

    d. orgasmic dysfunction.

d
Comprehension
Implementation
Promotion: Growth
and Development
Through the Life
Span

38-8   The most important thing for nurses to do in order to effectively help clients deal with sexual problems is to:

    a. take sex education classes.

    b. refer all of their questions to a physician.

    c. provide them with written information about sexual problems.

    d. become aware of their own attitudes about sexuality.

c
Application
Implementation
Promotion: Growth
and Development
Through the Life
Span

38-9   A 42-year-old man with diabetes is depressed because he has become impotent. How could a nurse help him improve his sexual functioning?

    a. Encourage self-stimulation.

    b. Suggest using the side-lying position for intercourse.

    c. Provide information about a penile prosthesis.

    d. Recommend having sex early in the morning.

c
Comprehension
Implementation
Promotion: Growth
and Development
Through the Life
Span

38-10   A 42-year-old man with diabetes is depressed because he has become impotent. How might he increase his level of sexual arousal?

    a. prolonged kissing

    b. breast stimulation

    c. genital stimulation

    d. alternating hugging and kissing

38-11   Which nursing diagnosis is defined as "the state in which one expresses concern regarding one's sexuality or experiences or is at risk of experiencing a change in sexual health?"

    a.   Altered Sexuality Patterns

    b.   Sexual Dysfunction

    c.   Body Image Disturbance

    d.   Altered Self-Concept

38-12   The outward expression of one's sense of sexuality or of what is perceived as appropriate with regard to one's sexuality (that is, 'acting like a man' or 'acting like a woman') is called:

    a   sexual stimulation.

    b.   gender-role behavior.

    c.   sexuality.

    d.   sexual health.

38-13   A condom worn during anal intercourse:

    a.   should not be lubricated because it may tear.

    b.   is unnecessary because one cannot become pregnant as a result of anal intercourse.

    c.   should not be used for subsequent vaginal intercourse.

    d.   will cause rectal tissue to tear and become infected.

38-14   Which form of sexual expression is unacceptable because it is illegal or infringes on the rights of others?

    a.   cunnilingus

    b.   anal intercourse

    c.   premature ejaculation

    d.   pedophilia

38-15   A client confides in the nurse that sex is not satisfying for her because her husband experiences premature ejaculation and refuses to see a counselor. The nurse should tell the client to continue trying to persuade her husband to see a therapist, but suggest that meanwhile:

    a.   she could take home some information about a penile implant.

    b.   the couple focus on communicating about sex and on enjoying touching without attempting intercourse.

    c.   they keep a clock by the bedside, and have the husband first attempt 15 seconds of penetration without ejaculation, then gradually increase the time.

    d.   the client try performing fellatio to increase the intensity of stimulation her husband experiences.

a
Knowledge
Analysis/Diagnosis
Promotion: Growth
and Development
Through the Life
Span

38-16   A woman who has never been able to achieve orgasm suffers from:

a. sexual dysfunction.

b. vulvodynia.

c. pedophilia.

d. impotence.

c
Comprehension
Implementation
Promotion: Growth
and Development
Through the Life
Span

38-38   When using the PLISSIT model of intervention to help clients with sexual problems, the nurse is implementing the 'P' portion of the model when she:

a. gives an accurate but concise explanation of what is normal and how the client's present situation or condition may affect sexual functioning.

b. uses specialized knowledge to suggest specific interventions that might be therapeutic (e.g., which sexual practices are safe following a heart attack).

c. acknowledges the client's sexual concerns and conveys the attitude that sexual needs are important to health and recovery.

d. refers the client to a clinical nurse-specialist or sex therapist.

b
Knowledge
Implementation
Promotion: Growth
and Development
Through the Life
Span

38-18   Which parts of the PLISSIT model can be effectively implemented by a nurse having basic and specific (but not specialized) knowledge on sexuality and sexual function and ways in which health problems can affect sexual function?

a. permission giving

b. permission giving and limited information

c. permission giving, limited information, and specific suggestions

d. permission giving, limited information, specific suggestions, and intensive therapy

c
Comprehension
Implementation
Promotion: Growth
and Development
Through the Life
Span

38-19   A couple wishes to prevent pregnancy, but their religion forbids them to use chemical, mechanical, or 'unnatural' methods. The nurse might suggest that they use:

a. an intrauterine device (IUD).

b. oral contraceptives.

c. coitus interruptus.

d. hormonal implants.

38-20   Some people object to the vaginal diaphragm and the vaginal sponge because:

  a. they must be inserted by a physician.

  b. they inhibit the spontaneity of intercourse and they are 'messy'.

  c. there are too many physical complications associated with their use.

  d. they must be removed immediately after intercourse in order to be effective.

38-21   Which sexual change occurs as a result of normal aging?

  a. Men experience erectile dysfunction.

  b. Men achieve erection and ejaculate more quickly.

  c. Women remain capable of orgasm but lose sexual desire after menopause.

  d. Women experience decreased vaginal lubrication and elasticity after menopause.

38-22   A nurse advises a client to practice 'safer sex' in order to avoid contracting AIDS and HIV. The client asks what is specifically meant by this term. The nurse should reply that safer sex means:

  a. having no exchanges of body fluids and no contact of body fluids with mucous membranes (e.g., oral, rectal, genital).

  b. wearing a condom for anal sexual intercourse.

  c. wearing a condom for anal or vaginal sexual intercourse.

  d. not engaging in cunnilingus or fellatio.

38-23   Which of the following statements is a sexual myth or misconception?

  a. It is not necessary for a woman to be orgasmic in order to become pregnant.

  b. Chronic alcoholism is associated with impotence.

  c. Masturbation is harmless.

  d. Alcohol is a sexual stimulant.

38-24   As the nurse is bathing a 40-year-old man who is paralyzed from the waist down, he reaches up and touches her on the breast. What should she do?

  a. Use direct eye contact and say firmly, "Don't do that."

  b. Pretend not to notice and continue the bed bath.

  c. Slap him and leave the room.

  d. Laugh and say, "You're feeling frisky today!"

d
Knowledge
Assessment
Promotion: Growth
and Development
Through the Life
Span

38-25   In the sexual response cycle, what is a *refractory period*?

a. a period of increasing muscle tension and excitement that occurs prior to orgasm

b. a period during which a man ejaculates

c. involuntary contractions of muscle groups throughout the body

d. a period during which the body will not respond to sexual stimulation

c
Comprehension
Implementation
Promotion: Growth
and Development
Through the Life
Span

38-26   Which birth control method also helps to prevent sexually transmitted diseases acquired through penile-vaginal intercourse?

a. diaphragm

b. oral contraceptives

c. condom

d. vaginal sponge

c
Application
Implementation
Promotion: Growth
and Development
Through the Life
Span

38-27   A man and woman at the nursing home have become very attached and want to have intimate sexual relations. Which nursing action would be most appropriate?

a. State that this is unacceptable behavior.

b. Tell them they will have to leave.

c. Provide them with uninterrupted time alone.

d. Ask them to state their plans in writing.

b
Application
Evaluation
Promotion: Growth
and Development
Through the Life
Span

38-28   Which statement indicates the client understands the teaching about reducing the discomfort of dysmenorrhea?

a. "I will avoid taking aspirin to make me feel better."

b. "A heating pad across my stomach for 15 minutes is helpful."

c. "Showering with cool or tepid water will feel best."

d. "Resting in bed for several hours will make me feel worse."

b
Application
Analysis/Diagnosis
Promotion: Growth
and Development
Through the Life
Span

38-29   Which nursing diagnosis would the nurse use for a client who indicates masturbation would make her crazy?

a. Anxiety related to bad feelings about masturbation

b. Knowledge Deficit: Normal Functions related to sexual myths

c. Risk for Sexual Dysfunction related to sexual ideas

d. Risk for Altered Sexuality Patterns related to concern for performance

38-30   In teaching a young man about testicular self-examination, it is important for the nurse to emphasize:

a.   checking the testicles consistently once a month.

b.   examining the testicles after a shower, when the body has cooled off.

c.   reporting any changes at his next annual physical.

d.   using a mirror to inspect for skin lesions on the scrotum.

38-31   Which question is appropriate for the nurse to ask a 38-year-old client who comes to the clinic for birth control pills?

a.   "Do your parents know you want this prescription?"

b.   "Are you familiar with safer sex practices?"

c.   "Do you think it is wise to be sexually active now?"

d.   "Have you already had sexual relations?"

a
Comprehension
Assessment
Psychosocial:
Coping and
Adaptation

39-1   A scale to assess and document a person's stressful life events is based upon the conceptualization of stress as a:

    a.   stimulus.

    b.   response.

    c.   transaction.

    d.   syndrome.

b
Comprehension
Psychosocial:
Coping and
Adaptation

39-2   Selye's general and local adaptation syndromes are examples of conceptualizing stress as a(n):

    a.   stimulus.

    b.   response.

    c.   transaction.

    d.   interaction.

a
Comprehension
Psychosocial:
Coping and
Adaptation

39-3   The two major homeostatic regulators of the body are the endocrine system and the:

    a.   autonomic nervous system.

    b.   sympathetic nervous system.

    c.   parasympathetic nervous system.

    d.   central nervous system.

c
Comprehension
Assessment
Physiological:
Physiological
Adaptation

39-4   An individual with a disease or tumor of which disease would probably be unable to mobilize an effective 'fight or flight' response to stressors because of insufficient epinephrine?

    a.   thyroid gland

    b.   pituitary gland

    c.   adrenal glands

    d.   parathyroid glands

d
Application
Assessment
Psychosocial:
Coping and
Adaptation

39-5   A 62-year-old client underwent a left radical mastectomy for carcinoma of the breast. She cried for days after the surgery, stating, "My life is ruined, I'll never be the same again. I wish I could die." Her roommate, a 24-year-old client, also underwent a radical mastectomy. The nurse should expect the younger client's reaction to be:

    a.   the same as the older woman's.

    b.   less severe than the older woman's.

    c.   more severe because she is younger.

    d.   different or the same.

b
Knowledge
Psychosocial:
Coping and
Adaptation

39-6   According to Hans Selye, stress is a(n):

a. event or set of circumstances causing a disrupted response.

b. nonspecific response of the body to any demanding situation.

c. transaction between the person and the environment.

d. stimulus threatening a person's homeostasis.

b
Comprehension
Analysis/Diagnosis
Physiological:
Physiological
Adaptation

39-7   A man cut his leg severely and it bled profusely until he applied a pressure dressing with his shirt. After a short period of time, a clot formed and the wound stopped bleeding. This physiological response, as described by Selye, is called the:

a. alarm reaction stage.

b. stage of resistance.

c. stage of exhaustion.

d. local adaptation syndrome.

a
Knowledge
Physiological:
Physiological
Adaptation

39-8   During times of stress, bronchial dilation takes place in response to secretion of:

a. epinephrine.

b. norepinephrine.

c. cortisone.

d. aldosterone.

a
Comprehension
Psychosocial:
Coping and
Adaptation

39-9   Coping with stress differs from adaptation to stress in that:

a. coping is a more immediate, short-term response to stress.

b. coping is a later response to stress.

c. adaptation is a more positive response to stress.

d. coping is a mode of resistance to stress.

b
Application
Analysis/Diagnosis
Psychosocial:
Coping and
Adaptation

39-10   A student is preparing to take her final examination in Nursing 101. She feels tense and nervous, and her respiratory and pulse rates are increased. Which level of anxiety is she experiencing?

a. mild

b. moderate

c. severe

d. panic

c
Knowledge
Promotion: Growth
and Development
Through the Life
Span

39-11   Anger is a feeling of strong displeasure which is:

a. an unhealthy emotional state, but socially acceptable.

b. an internal emotion not displayed or expressed openly.

c. a positive emotion and a sign of emotional maturity.

d. never communicated until the tension is discharged.

a
Comprehension
Implementation
Psychosocial:
Coping and
Adaptation

39-12 In order to be constructive, verbal expressions of anger must be:

a. communicated clearly.

b. made without raising the voice.

c. avoided until the feeling subsides.

d. given only indirectly, as suggestions.

b
Application
Analysis/Diagnosis
Psychosocial:
Coping and
Adaptation

39-13 A parent says to a child, "Stop right now! *I get very upset when you leave your toys in the middle of the floor.*" The italicized portion of the parent's comment represents an expression of:

a. aggression.

b. anger.

c. hostility.

d. violence.

a
Knowledge
Assessment
Psychosocial:
Coping and
Adaptation

39-14 Which example indicates a cognitive response to stress?

a. daydreaming

b. sleeping

c. holding and touching

d. laughing

a
Application
Assessment
Psychosocial:
Coping and
Adaptation

39-15 Certain physiologic changes in a client seem to indicate that she is experiencing a high degree of stress. Which intervention would best enable the nurse to determine the amount of anxiety or psychological stress the client is experiencing?

a. Say, "You seem worried about something. Would it help to talk about it?"

b. Ask the client to complete a Mood States Profile.

c. Ask, "Do you think your illness is serious?"

d. Call a significant other to support her and reduce her anxiety.

a
Application
Analysis/Diagnosis
Psychosocial:
Coping and
Adaptation

39-16 Physiologic and psychologic assessment indicate that a client is experiencing a high degree of stress. She states that her family won't be able to visit until the weekend because they don't have transportation. When the nurse tries to involve her in planning her care, she says, "I don't know what to do. I can't make decisions without my family. I'm afraid and I'm mad at them for not finding a way to get here!" Based on this data, an appropriate nursing diagnosis for this client is:

a. Ineffective Individual Coping related to absence of support system.

b. Ineffective Individual Coping related to multiple life changes.

c. Ineffective Family Coping related to prolonged illness.

d. Ineffective Family Coping related to unexpressed anger.

a
Comprehension
Planning
Psychosocial:
Coping and
Adaptation

39-17 The overall goals for clients experiencing stress-related responses are to decrease anxiety and fear and to:

a. increase their coping abilities.

b. enable them to function independently.

c. promote social interaction.

d. prevent expressions of anger.

c
Application
Planning
Psychosocial:
Coping and
Adaptation

39-18 A male client is experiencing much stress since he has been hospitalized, and his support system is very limited because he has just moved to this country without his family. What would be the best intervention to help him cope with his stress?

a. Keep him busy so his time goes by quickly.

b. Provide as much privacy as possible.

c. Provide for adequate rest and relaxation.

d. If he does not express his feelings, ask questions until he does so.

d
Knowledge
Psychosocial:
Coping and
Adaptation

39-19 All adaptive responses have common characteristics. One such characteristic is that they:

a. are the same for all people.

b. provide short-term relief from stress.

c. are unlimited.

d. may be inadequate or excessive.

b
Knowledge
Analysis/Diagnosis
Psychosocial:
Coping and
Adaptation

39-20 Which nursing diagnosis is defined as "the state in which the individual experiences feelings of uneasiness and activation of the autonomic nervous system in response to a vague, nonspecific threat?"

a. Fear

b. Anxiety

c. Ineffective Individual Coping

d. Decisional Conflict

a
Comprehension
Implementation
Psychosocial:
Coping and
Adaptation

39-21 For the nurse to assist the client in reducing anxiety, what is an essential first step?

a. The client must recognize that he/she is anxious.

b. The client must discuss common fears and concerns.

c. The nurse must explain the source of the anxiety.

d. The nurse must demonstrate effective communication skills.

d
Comprehension
Implementation
Psychosocial:
Coping and
Adaptation

39-22   Which general nursing intervention would be most effective in reducing a client's anger?

a. providing reassurance

b. offering advice

c. giving an aggressive response

d. asking relevant questions

d
Comprehension
Implementation
Psychosocial:
Coping and
Adaptation

39-23   Which activity is an effective stress management strategy for nurses?

a. Organize tasks more efficiently so you do not need to delegate to others.

b. Avoid colleagues who are ventilating their concerns or feelings.

c. Learn to be agreeable and helpful; never say no to a colleague.

d. Accept what can't be changed, including your own limitations.

c
Comprehension
Assessment
Psychosocial:
Coping and
Adaptation

39-24   Which behavior is characteristic of someone who is coping well?

a. sleeps 4 or 5 hours a night

b. drinks alcohol to relieve stress

c. sets aside 30 minutes a day to exercise

d. has no hobbies

b
Application
Analysis/Diagnosis
Psychosocial:
Coping and
Adaptation

39-25   A nursing student who is very fearful of injections is preparing to give her first intramuscular injection. She states she can't do it because she knows the client is very fearful of injections. The student is using a defense mechanism called:

a. rationalization.

b. projection.

c. denial.

d. compensation.

b
Application
Implementation
Psychosocial:
Coping and
Adaptation

39-26   Which intervention should the nurse teach a client who has been under a lot of stress to use to reduce the effects of stress?

a. Think about problems and feelings.

b. Reduce coffee to one cup in the morning.

c. Eat high-calorie foods to increase energy level.

d. Try to handle all tasks each day.

39-27   A nurse has been working on a cardiac stepdown unit for three years. In the last two months he has been absent once a week with various ailments. When he does work, he spends a lot of time complaining about the work load to his colleagues. Which coping strategy would be most appropriate for this nurse?

    a.   Refuse to care for additional clients on his shift.

    b.   Continue to smoke as it makes him less nervous.

    c.   Circulate a petition about the unfairness of the work load.

    d.   Form a support group with the other nurses on the unit.

39-28   A woman has been caring for her sister for the last six months without relief from other family members who live in another state. Lately she has been unable to sleep at night and very tearful. Which nursing diagnosis is appropriate?

    a.   Anxiety related to demands of caring for sister

    b. Ineffective Denial related to sleeplessness

    c.   Defensive Coping related to strain of caring for sister

    d.   Caregiver Role Strain related to lack of support in caring for sister

39-29   Which statement indicates the client understands the teaching about methods of minimizing stress in her life?

    a.   "It will help if I do everything myself so my partner can relax."

    b. "Skipping lunch will give me more time to run errands and may help me lose weight."

    c.   "My partner has agreed to watch the children when I take bubble baths."

    d.   "I must straighten up the living areas every night before going to bed."

d
Application
Analysis/Diagnosis
Psychosocial:
Coping and
Adaptation

40-1   Which one of the following individuals most likely exhibits dysfunctional grieving?

     a.   someone who cries for several hours at his partner's funeral

     b.   someone who visits her mother's grave repeatedly in the first year following the death

     c.   someone who cannot acknowledge the loss of a loved one to others

     d.   someone who separates from interactions with others for prolonged periods

b
Comprehension
Planning
Psychosocial:
Coping and
Adaptation

40-2   The nurse recognizes that more even than the fear of death itself, older adults fear:

     a.   nausea.

     b.   loss of control.

     c.   the cost of terminal care.

     d.   the unknown.

d
Application
Analysis/Diagnosis
Psychosocial:
Coping and
Adaptation

40-3   A client is going to have his leg amputated tomorrow. He has been grieving for the past week. Which of the following best describes what he is experiencing?

     a.   dysfunctional grief

     b.   perceived loss

     c.   bereavement

     d.   anticipatory grief

a
Knowledge
Assessment
Psychosocial:
Coping and
Adaptation

40-4   The subjective response of an individual to the death of a significant other is called:

     a.   bereavement.

     b.   grief.

     c.   mourning.

     d.   crisis.

d
Knowledge
Assessment
Promotion: Growth
and Development
Through the Life
Span

40-5   In which of the following age ranges is the acceptance of one's own mortality a characteristic of the concept of death?

     a.   9 to 12 years

     b.   12 to 18 years

     c.   18 to 45 years

     d.   45 to 65 years

b
Knowledge
Assessment
Physiological:
Physiological
Adaptation

40-6   Which of the following is a clinical sign of imminent death?

    a. flat encephalogram

    b. sensory impairment

    c. muscle rigidity

    d. unconsciousness

c
Knowledge
Physiological:
Physiological
Adaptation

40-7   In caring for a dying client, it is important for the nurse to act with the knowledge that the last sense lost in dying is thought to be:

    a. sight.

    b. smell.

    c. hearing.

    d. touch.

c
Application
Analysis/Diagnosis
Psychosocial:
Coping and
Adaptation

40-8   Your client died at the beginning of the day shift. The client's daughter told the nurse that she was relieved and glad they had discussed her mother's wishes for funeral arrangements the previous evening. These statements suggest the daughter is in a state of:

    a. closed awareness.

    b. mutual pretense.

    c. open awareness.

    d. social isolation.

a
Comprehension
Analysis/Diagnosis
Psychosocial:
Coping and
Adaptation

40-9   In providing support for a bereaved client, the nurse needs to be aware that grieving is:

    a. essential for good mental and physical health after a loss.

    b. best carried out in solitude.

    c. socially unacceptable in present-day American culture.

    d. detrimental to emotional well-being.

c
Application
Implementation
Physiological:
Physiological
Adaptation

40-10   After a client died, the physician agreed that the body could remain on the unit for as long as the family wished to view it or until rigor mortis began. The nurse should inform the family that they can expect to remain with the client for about:

    a. 30 to 60 minutes.

    b. 60 to 90 minutes.

    c. 2 to 4 hours.

    d. 4 to 6 hours.

d Knowledge Psychosocial: Coping and Adaptation	40-11	According to Elizabeth Kubler-Ross, the five stages or phases of dying are denial, _____, bargaining, depression, and acceptance. a. shock b. restitution c. protest d. anger
a Application Implementation Psychosocial: Coping and Adaptation	40-12	The terminally ill client states to the nurse, "I'm just not ready to go." The most appropriate response by the nurse would be: a. "Tell me more about what you mean when you say that you're not ready." b. "You're not ready to go where?" c. "Oh, there's really nothing to be afraid of. Dying is a natural process." d. "I can understand that. Most people don't want to die."
a Application Analysis/Diagnosis Psychosocial: Coping and Adaptation	33.13	After a biopsy, the client tells his physician that if the mass is malignant, he wants to know, but he does not want any further treatment or his family to know. The client is exhibiting a state of: a. closed awareness. b. open awareness. c. partial awareness. d. mutual pretense.
c Application Planning Psychosocial: Coping and Adaptation	40-14	After a biopsy, the client tells his physician that if the mass is malignant, he wants to know, but he does not want any further treatment or his family to know. A major nursing responsibility in caring for the client would be to: a. convince him to tell his family. b. suggest he consider treatment options. c. support his decisions regarding care. d. contact his family so they can help him.
c Comprehension Psychosocial: Coping and Adaptation	40-15	Grieving provides a bereaved individual the opportunity to: a. obliterate unpleasant thoughts about the deceased. b. avoid painful memories and hold positive ones. c. feel free from emotional bondage to the deceased. d. postpone making new relationships.

b
Comprehension
Analysis/Diagnosis
Psychosocial:
Coping and
Adaptation

40-16 When a change in health status requires modification in lifestyle that a person is unable to make, a likely nursing diagnosis is:

a. Body Image Disturbance.

b. Impaired Adjustment.

c. Altered Self-Concept.

d. Anxiety.

a
Comprehension
Planning
Psychosocial:
Coping and
Adaptation

40-17 For clients in the end stage of terminal illness, what can hospice care provide?

a. meet the client's physical, emotional, social, and economic needs.

b. ease or reduce the effect of a disease and temporarily ease pain, but not cure the disease.

c. care for all dying clients at home until death

d. one health professional to care for all the client's needs

b
Knowledge
Psychosocial:
Coping and
Adaptation

40-18 Which type of services are created especially to provide holistic care for clients in the end stage of terminal illness?

a. hospitalization

b. hospice care

c. extended care facility

d. convalescent care

a
Knowledge
Implementation
Psychosocial:
Coping and
Adaptation

40-19 In order for nurses to effectively provide spiritual health care, it is most important for them to:

a. evaluate their own ability to interact supportively in this area.

b. enhance the client's body image.

c. provide accurate information and education.

d. assist the client to identify spiritual concerns.

b
Knowledge
Assessment
Promotion: Growth
and Development
Through the Life
Span

40-20 The earliest age at which most persons accept death as being irreversible is:

a. 3 years old.

b. 5 years old.

c. 9 years old.

d. 12 years old.

a
Application
Implementation
Psychosocial:
Coping and
Adaptation

40-21 Which of the following interventions would best help to maintain a dying client's dignity and sense of self-worth?

a. Allow the client to make choices and set her own timetable for scheduled activities.

b. Suggest that the client die quietly at home in a familiar environment.

c. Have other terminally ill individuals visit the client.

d. Schedule as much uninterrupted quiet time as possible for the client to reflect on her past.

c
Knowledge
Safety: Management
of Care

40-22 The legal document that specifies the health care wishes of a terminally ill client is the:

a. Patient Self-Determination Act.

b. durable power of attorney for health care.

c. living will.

d. no code order.

b
Application
Assessment
Physiological:
Physiological
Adaptation

41-1   Which of the following clients is most at risk for developing complications of immobility?

     a.   a 30-year-old with a fractured ankle

     b.   an 80-year-old with a fractured hip

     c.   a 2-year-old with a burned hand

     d.   a 42-year-old who is one day post abdominal surgery

b
Knowledge
Physiological:
Physiological
Adaptation

41-2   The term *catabolism* refers to:

     a.   protein synthesis.

     b.   protein breakdown.

     c.   lack of appetite.

     d.   abnormally small amounts of protein in the blood.

a
Comprehension
Assessment
Physiological:
Physiological
Adaptation

41-3   Which of the following groups of physiologic alterations is frequently a result of immobility?

     a.   bony demineralization, increased heart rate, venous pooling, decreased vital capacity

     b.   increased ciliary movement, decreased catabolism, positive calcium balance, diuresis

     c.   urinary stasis, decreased heart rate, increased intestinal motility, venous pooling

     d.   constipation, bony demineralization, increased secretion of digestive juices, nitrogen retention

c
Knowledge
Assessment
Physiological:
Reduction of Risk
Potential

41-4   A therapeutic effect of bedrest is that it:

     a.   facilitates lung expansion.

     b.   increases peristalsis.

     c.   reduces the oxygen needs of cells.

     d.   enhances protein anabolism.

a
Application
Evaluation
Physiological:
Physiological
Adaptation

41-5   A client is in traction and confined to bed following an automobile accident. Which of the following responses would allow the nurse to conclude that the client's psychoneurologic system has not been affected by her immobility?

     a.   The client is explaining to her husband how to solve a problem that has occurred with their baby sitter.

     b.   The client's appetite is unchanged since her hospital admission.

     c.   The client is somewhat withdrawn and does not initiate conversation.

     d.   When trying to brush her teeth and perform other ADLs, the client is frustrated easily.

41-6 A client turns the sole of the foot outward (away from the midline of the body). This is called:

    a. external rotation.

    b. dorsiflexion.

    c. eversion.

    d. inversion.

41-7 Movement of a limb away from the midline of the body is called:

    a. abduction.

    b. adduction.

    c. flexion.

    d. extension.

41-8 A standing client moves the palm of his hand from a posterior to an anterior position. This is called:

    a. eversion.

    b. palmar rotation.

    c. supination.

    d. anterior rotation.

41-9 A 70-year-old client has been hospitalized with a medical diagnosis of rheumatoid arthritis. She has been treated by her physician at home on bedrest for the past three weeks. When performing the initial assessment, which of the following data should be of primary concern to the nurse?

    a. elevated white blood cell count and elevated hematocrit

    b. increased heart rate, dependent edema, and chest pain

    c. joint pain on movement, joint redness, and swelling

    d. weight loss of five pounds and loss of appetite

41-10 An assessment of a client's *ADL* should include an observation of:

    a. vital signs.

    b. range of joint motion.

    c. intake and output.

    d. ability to bathe and dress.

41-11 Which of the following data provides the best assessment of a client's activity tolerance?

    a. vital capacity and breath sounds

    b. degrees of joint flexibility

    c. muscle strength and coordination

    d. vital signs before, during, and after an activity

c
Comprehension
Evaluation
Physiological: Basic
Care and Comfort

41-12   The doctor has ordered progressive ambulation for a client who has been on bedrest. When the nurse assists him out of bed for the first time, the client becomes dizzy when he sits up. The nurse should:

a.   continue to get him up slowly.

b.   suggest that he take deep breaths.

c.   lower the head of the bed until symptoms subside.

d.   inform the doctor that the client is not ready to ambulate.

a
Application
Planning
Physiological:
Physiological
Adaptation

41-13   An immobilized client complains of pain in her right calf when moving her foot or leg. The nurse notes edema, weak peripheral pulses, and cool skin on the right leg. The nurse should:

a.   notify the physician.

b.   massage the calf.

c.   encourage the client to ambulate more.

d.   encourage the client to lie on her left side more.

b
Knowledge
Implementation
Physiological:
Reduction of Risk
Potential

41-14   Passive range of motion should be performed:

a.   to the point of discomfort.

b.   to the point of slight resistance.

c.   with the client sitting up.

d.   on limbs that the client can exercise unassisted.

b
Comprehension
Analysis/Diagnosis
Physiological:
Physiological
Adaptation

41-15   A client has dyspnea and fatigue even when at rest. An appropriate nursing diagnosis label for her is:

a.   Activity Intolerance: Level I.

b.   Activity Intolerance: Level IV.

c.   Impaired Physical Mobility: Level I.

d.   Impaired Physical Mobility: Level IV.

c
Comprehension
Analysis/Diagnosis
Physiological:
Physiological
Adaptation

41-16   A client must use a walker to ambulate. Otherwise, he needs no special assistance. An appropriate nursing diagnosis label for the client is:

a.   Activity Intolerance: Level I.

b.   Activity Intolerance: Level IV.

c.   Impaired Physical Mobility: Level I.

d.   Impaired Physical Mobility: Level IV.

d
Application
Planning
Promotion:
Prevention and Early
Detection of Disease

41-17   A nurse is helping develop an exercise program for a healthy 20-year-old client. The client is a driver for a package delivery company. The nurse should advise the client to:

a.   begin her exercise sessions with the most strenuous activity and end with the least strenuous.

b.   see her physician before initiating an exercise program.

c.   exercise alone to avoid distraction.

d.   end her exercise sessions with a five-minute cool-down period of light activity.

c
Comprehension
Physiological:
Physiological
Adaptation

41-18   Which of the following is an immediate effect of exercise on the heart?

a.   It reduces the resting heart rate.

b.   It reduces the heart rate with exertion.

c.   It increases cardiac output and systolic blood pressure.

d.   It increases the size of the heart muscle.

b
Comprehension
Implementation
Physiological: Basic
Care and Comfort

41-19   Which of the following demonstrates wheelchair safety?

a.   The nurse pushes the client face-forward ahead of her into the elevator.

b.   The nurse raises the footplates before transferring the client into the wheelchair.

c.   The nurse positions the client as far forward as possible on the wheelchair seat.

d.   The nurse positions the chair ahead of her when going down a ramp.

d
Knowledge
Planning
Physiological:
Reduction of Risk
Potential

41-20   For a client with a nursing diagnosis of Impaired Mobility related to bedrest, weakness, and traction apparatus, what is the rationale for maintaining the client in good body alignment in the bed?

a.   It increases body strength and muscle mass.

b.   It decreases protein catabolism and improves nitrogen balance.

c.   It minimizes the workload of the heart by preventing Valsalva maneuvers.

d.   It reduces the musculoskeletal strain and enhances lung expansion.

a
Comprehension
Planning
Physiological:
Reduction of Risk
Potential

41-21   A 68-year-old widow does ironing to supplement her Social Security
         income. She suffers from lordosis and has come to the doctor's office
         complaining of severe low back pain and fatigue. Which of the following
         interventions would be most helpful to her?

         a.   Suggest that she elevate one foot on a stool when standing at the
              ironing board.
         b.   Explain the potential for injuring her back if she continues to take in
              ironing.
         c.   Prescribe aspirin to decrease discomfort and inflammation.
         d.   Have her take frequent short naps to reduce her fatigue.

a
Knowledge
Implementation
Promotion:
Prevention and Early
Detection of Disease

41-22   What are the three basic concepts that must be considered in achieving
         good body mechanics?

         a.   body alignment, balance, and coordinated body movement
         b.   body alignment, inertia, and gravity
         c.   center of gravity, balance, and base of support
         d.   coordinated body movement, strength, and posture

d
Comprehension
Implementation
Physiological:
Reduction of Risk
Potential

41-23   For a client on bedrest, a footboard creates pressure against the sole of the
         foot, eliciting a reflexive contraction of the extensor muscles of the lower
         legs. The primary importance of this intervention is to:

         a.   maintain the muscle strength of the lower extremities.
         b.   prevent contractures of the lower extremities.
         c.   give the client better stability for changing positions in bed.
         d.   maintain postural tonus for the time when the client again resumes an
              upright position.

b
Knowledge
Assessment
Physiological:
Physiological
Adaptation

41-24   A permanent shortening of a muscle and the eventual shortening of
         associated ligaments and tendons is known as:

         a.   dysplasia.
         b.   a contracture.
         c.   kyphoscoliosis.
         d.   a pathologic fracture.

c
Comprehension
Planning
Physiological:
Reduction of Risk
Potential

41-25   A client's activity level order has been changed from bedrest to 'bedside
         chair tid'. Before attempting to ambulate the client to the chair, the nurse
         determines that the chair seat seems too low for his height. What can the
         nurse do to alleviate this problem?

         a.   Wait until an appropriate chair is available before moving the client.
         b.   Allow the client to remain in the chair for only five minutes at a time.
         c.   Place pillows in the chair seat to make it higher.
         d.   Place one pillow between the client's back and the chair and one
              under his thighs.

a
Knowledge
Evaluation
Physiological:
Reduction of Risk
Potential

41-26 After helping the client from the bed to a bedside chair, the nurse evaluates his sitting position. Which of the following indicates correct alignment?

   a. popliteal spaces away from the edge of the chair
   b. head flexed forward slightly
   c. knees extended
   d. soles of the feet plantar flexed

b
Knowledge
Implementation
Physiological:
Reduction of Risk
Potential

41-27 After helping a client to a bedside chair, the nurse should caution him about some common problems of sitting, such as slouching and:

   a. tilting his pelvis.
   b. crossing his legs.
   c. leaning forward.
   d. flexing his feet.

c
Comprehension
Implementation
Physiological:
Reduction of Risk
Potential

41-28 A client has been hospitalized with medical diagnoses of osteoporosis and compression fracture of the lumbar spine. Her physician has ordered complete bedrest and meeting with a dietician for nutritional counseling. The dietician will most likely focus on helping the client to understand the importance of:

   a. vitamin D in her diet and from the sun.
   b. reducing her calorie and fat intake.
   c. an adequate calcium intake.
   d. sufficient protein intake.

a
Application
Analysis/Diagnosis
Physiological:
Physiological
Adaptation

41-29 A client has been hospitalized with medical diagnoses of osteoporosis and compression fracture of the lumbar spine. She complains of lower back pain. Her physician has ordered complete bedrest. Based on this data, one appropriate nursing diagnosis for the client would be:

   a. Pain related to back injury secondary to osteoporosis.
   b. Risk for Injury related to poor alignment and bedrest.
   c. Activity Intolerance related to back injury.
   d. Altered Nutrition: Less than Body Requirements related to poor dietary habits.

a
Knowledge
Planning
Physiological:
Reduction of Risk
Potential

41-30 A client complaining of lower back pain has been hospitalized with medical diagnoses of osteoporosis and compression fracture of the lumbar spine. Her physician has ordered complete bedrest. The nurse plans a systematic 24-hour schedule for frequent position changes. The rationale for this intervention is to:

a. prevent skin breakdown.
b. prevent flexion contractures.
c. relieve back pain.
d. minimize muscle fatigue and promote good alignment.

c
Comprehension
Planning
Physiological:
Reduction of Risk
Potential

41-31 When turning a client to the left side-lying position, the nurse should use supportive devices in order to:

a. prevent skin breakdown.
b. allow the client's top leg to rest on the lower leg.
c. maintain the natural alignment of the body.
d. prevent stasis of urine in the kidneys.

b
Knowledge
Analysis/Diagnosis
Physiological: Basic
Care and Comfort

41-32 The nurse sees that the head of a client's bed is elevated about 60° and her knees are slightly elevated. The nurse appropriately charts the client to be in which of the following positions?

a. supine
b. Fowler's
c. Sims'
d. prone

b
Comprehension
Planning
Physiological: Basic
Care and Comfort

41-33 A client is to receive a backrub to help her relax. The best position for this procedure is:

a. supine.
b. prone.
c. Fowler's.
d. recumbent.

b
Knowledge
Assessment
Safety: Safety and
Infection Control

41-34 What is the most common serious mobility problem for hospitalized clients?

a. burns
b. falls
c. muscle strain
d. contractures

41-35   The major work-related threat to nurses' health is:

a. drug abuse.

b. depression.

c. back injury.

d. falls.

41-36   A nurse weighs 125 pounds. The box of sterile instruments she is supposed to transport to the treatment room weighs 50 pounds. What would be the appropriate method for lifting the box?

a. She should bend at the knees, keep her back straight, and lift the box.

b. She should seek help from another person before moving the box.

c. She should use a mechanical device to move the box.

d. She should return to the unit and ask a male employee to transport the box for her.

41-37   Which of the following is a correct principle of body mechanics?

a. The narrower the base of support and the lower the center of gravity, the greater the stability of the nurse.

b. Stooping with the hips flexed, knees straight, and trunk in good alignment distributes the workload among the largest and strongest muscle groups.

c. Facing in the opposite direction of movement prevents abnormal twisting of the spine.

d. Moving an object on a level surface requires less effort than moving the same object up an inclined surface.

41-38   When helping a client to move up in bed, the nurse should:

a. elevate the head of the bed 15°.

b. push rather than pull.

c. lower the entire bed as far as it will go.

d. use his or her own body weight in a rocking motion.

41-39   Which of the following normal developmental variations in body alignment is found in toddlers?

a. marked lumbar lordosis and protruding abdomen

b. inversion of the feet

c. a forward-leaning, stooped posture

d. straight legs with toes pointed straight ahead

c
Comprehension
Planning
Physiological: Basic
Care and Comfort

41-40 A client is to be discharged using crutches to assist with ambulation. Which of the following would be a correct outcome to use as an evaluation criterion?

a. When crutch-walking, the client's body weight is supported by her axillae.

b. When the client is standing upright with her hands on the handgrips, her elbows are slightly flexed.

c. When the client uses the tripod position, she places the crutch tips 15 cm to the side of each foot and about midway between the heel and great toe.

d. When ascending the stairs, the client places her weight on her strong leg while moving her crutches and affected leg onto the next step.

c
Application
Implementation
Physiological: Basic
Care and Comfort

41-41 A client's nursing diagnosis is Impaired Physical Mobility. The etiology is arthritis with severe right knee edema. What would be a nursing intervention for this diagnosis?

a. Active ROM to affected joint three BID.

b. Place pillow beneath right knee.

c. Limit weight bearing on right knee.

d. Ambulate frequently.

b
Comprehension
Implementation
Physiological:
Reduction of Risk
Potential

41-42 The nurse is instructing a client in traction to perform isometric exercises. This type of exercise will:

a. prevent contractures

b. maintain muscle strength

c. decrease heart rate

d. improve cardiorespiratory function

b
Application
Assessment
Physiological:
Reduction of Risk
Potential

41-43 Before a nurse transfers a client from bed to wheelchair he needs to assess the client's:

a. vital signs.

b. physical and mental capabilities.

c. height and weight.

d. position sense.

41-44 A nurse has provided a client with information on controlling the weakness and dizziness (postural hypotension) he feels when getting out of bed in the morning. What statement by the client indicates that the nurse's teaching has been effective?

    a. "I should sleep with my head flat, without any pillows."

    b. "I should keep my legs in a dependent position when sitting."

    c. "I should avoid sudden changes in position and take my time getting out of bed."

    d. "I should take a hot shower and shave right after I get out of bed in the morning."

41-45 A client has left lower extremity weakness. To evaluate the client's ability to use a walker, what should the nurse observe the client doing?

    a. moving the walker and the affected extremity 6 inches ahead, then moving the unaffected extremity while the weight is supported by the arms and affected extremity

    b. moving the walker and the unaffected extremity 6 inches ahead, then moving the affected extremity forward

    c. moving the walker ahead about 6 inches while bearing weight on both extremities and then walking with the arms pulling the walker

    d. moving the walker 12 inches forward while bearing weight on both extremities, then moving the unaffected extremity followed by the affected extremity toward the walker

42

a
Comprehension
Analysis/Diagnosis
Promotion:
Prevention and Early
Detection of Disease

42-1 Sleep is considered to be a state of:

a. consciousness with perception of the environment decreased with response to meaningful stimuli.

b. consciousness with no perception of the environment and no response to stimuli.

c. unconsciousness with perception of strong stimuli only.

d. unconsciousness with heightened perception of external stimuli.

b
Application
Implementation
Psychosocial:
Coping and
Adaptation

42-2 A client was admitted to ICU after a heart attack. He is upset because there is no telephone in his room and he states that he must make some business calls at once. How can the nurse best meet the client's needs at this time?

a. Ask the physician to prescribe a sedative.

b. Provide him with a telephone to make the calls.

c. Offer to make the phone calls for him.

d. Inform him that he needs to rest and can make the calls in a day or two.

d
Application
Analysis/Diagnosis
Psychosocial:
Coping and
Adaptation

42-3 A client is going to have a cardiac catheterization in the morning. Although it is late at night, she is having difficulty falling asleep. The appropriate nursing diagnosis for the client is:

a. Insomnia related to fear.

b. Fear related to diagnostic test.

c. Anxiety related to sleep pattern disturbance.

d. Sleep Pattern Disturbance related to anxiety.

d
Knowledge
Assessment
Promotion:
Prevention and Early
Detection of Disease

42-4 During which stage of NREM sleep would you expect a client to be most difficult to arouse?

a. Stage I

b. Stage II

c. Stage III

d. Stage IV

42-5   A client does not sleep during the six days she is hospitalized. After being discharged, she is very tired on her first night at home. How would you expect this to affect her sleep cycle?

    a.   Dreams will be prolonged.

    b.   REM sleep will predominate.

    c.   REM sleep cycles will last five minutes during the early portion of sleep.

    d.   Stage IV NREM sleep will last 30 minutes during each cycle.

42-6   A 72-year-old client has a hospital room located at the far end of the hall, away from the nurses' station. She is concerned that no one will hear her if she gets sick during the night. In order to alleviate her anxiety, the most appropriate nursing intervention would be to:

    a.   demonstrate to her how the call bell system works.

    b.   suggest that she have a family member stay with her.

    c.   have her transferred to a room close to the nurses' station.

    d.   tell her that a nurse will look in on her at least every two hours.

42-.7   It is now midnight and a client is still unable to fall asleep. What should the nurse do to help him sleep?

    a.   Bring him a glass of iced tea.

    b.   Suggest that he walk up and down the hall until he becomes tired enough to sleep.

    c.   Open the window or turn down the thermostat to bring the room temperature to below 50° F.

    d.   Make sure that his bed linen is wrinkle-free, and offer him a back massage.

42-8   Since being in the hospital, a client has taken her baths in the morning according to hospital routine; however, at home, she always took a warm bath just before going to bed. Now she has developed difficulty sleeping. What should the nurse do to help the client sleep better?

    a.   Rub her back for 15 minutes before she retires.

    b.   Offer her warm milk and crackers at 9:00 P.M.

    c.   Allow her to take her bath in the evening.

    d.   Ask her physician for a P.M. sleeping medication.

42-9 A client is scheduled to have vital signs taken at midnight, to receive medications at 1:00 A.M. and 5:00 A.M., and to have blood drawn for lab work at 6:30 A.M. How should the nurse provide periods of undisturbed sleep for the client?

a. Ask the lab to draw his blood at 5:00 A.M. instead of 6:30 A.M.

b. Ask the physician to change the times for medication administration.

c. Give the 1:00 A.M. dose of medication and take the midnight vital signs both at 12:30 A.M.

d. Delay the 5:00 A.M. dose of medication until the lab draws his blood at 6:30 A.M.

42-10 A 32-year-old mother of two has just returned home from the hospital with her new baby. She has been getting up every three hours during the night to feed him. What effect will this have on her sleep cycle?

a. It will increase REM sleep.

b. It will decrease REM sleep.

c. It will increase stage IV NREM sleep.

d. It will decrease stage IV NREM sleep.

42-11 In which age group is stage IV sleep markedly decreased or absent?

a. newborn

b. toddler

c. young adult

d. elderly adult

42-12 The most common sleep disorder is:

a. insomnia.

b. hypersomnia.

c. narcolepsy.

d. sleep apnea.

42-13 A six-year-old client has enlarged tonsils from frequent streptococcal infections. How might these enlarged tonsils affect her sleep?

a. cause sleep apnea

b. increase REM sleep

c. precipitate narcolepsy

d. decrease stage IV NREM sleep

b
Knowledge
Analysis/Diagnosis
Physiological:
Physiological
Adaptation

42-14   A young adult client suffers from attacks of overwhelming sleepiness that occur during the day. This type of sleepiness is called:

a.   insomnia.

b.   narcolepsy.

c.   parasomnia.

d.   hypersomnia.

d
Comprehension
Implementation
Physiological: Basic
Care and Comfort

42-15   A client is discouraged because his two-year-old daughter always resists going to sleep at her bedtime. What should he do to promote his daughter's sleep?

a.   Eliminate her afternoon nap.

b.   Offer her a bedtime snack.

c.   Wake her 30 minutes earlier each morning.

d.   Maintain a consistent pre-bedtime ritual.

a
Knowledge
Physiological: Basic
Care and Comfort

42-16   What is the relationship between the reticular activating system (RAS) and sleep?

a.   The RAS maintains wakefulness in the cerebral cortex.

b.   The RAS ends stimuli from the cerebral cortex to the body.

c.   The RAS suppresses brain centers.

d.   The RAS controls the body's biorhythms.

b
Knowledge
Assessment
Physiological: Basic
Care and Comfort

42-17   Dreaming occurs:

a.   within 10 minutes after falling asleep.

b.   during REM sleep.

c.   during stage I NREM sleep.

d.   in all stages of sleep.

c
Knowledge
Assessment
Physiological: Basic
Care and Comfort

42-18   Physiological changes during sleep include increased:

a.   pulse rate.

b.   basal metabolic rate.

c.   activity of the gastrointestinal tract.

d.   tonus of the skeletal muscles.

a
Knowledge
Assessment
Physiological: Basic
Care and Comfort

42-19   Which of the following is a symptom of NREM deprivation, but *not* of REM deprivation?

a.   excessive sleepiness

b.   emotional liability

c.   excitability

d.   confusion and suspiciousness

a
Application
Analysis/Diagnosis
Safety: Safety and
Infection Control

42-20   A nursing diagnosis of Risk for Injury: Falls would be appropriate for a client with which of the following parasomnias?

a.   somnambulism

b.   nocturnal enuresis

c.   nocturnal erections

d.   bruxism

b
Application
Assessment
Physiological:
Physiological
Adaptation

42-21   A client is being admitted to the medical unit with a diagnosis of upper gastrointestinal bleeding due to a gastric ulcer. During her admission nursing history she tells the nurse she hasn't been getting any sleep at night and she is so tired. Based on her history, what should the nurse investigate?

a.   her diet, with particular attention to the evening meal

b.   if pain is the reason she is waking up

c.   her environment

d.   her history of urinary tract infections

a
Comprehension
Assessment
Physiological:
Pharmacological and
Parenteral Therapies

42-22   A client has been receiving meperidine hydrochloride around the clock for pain. This medication affects sleep by:

a.   decreasing REM sleep.

b.   increasing REM sleep.

c.   increasing NREM sleep.

d.   increasing sleep cycles.

b
Application
Assessment
Physiological: Basic
Care and Comfort

42-23   A client presents to the clinic with chief complaint of fatigue and inability to sleep at night. Which nursing physical assessment findings would support the client's statement?

a.   attentiveness with good posture

b.   puffy red eyes and irritability

c.   patient, understanding, and quiet demeanor

d.   coordinated, rapid speech

c
Application
Implementation
Physiological: Basic
Care and Comfort

42-24   The first nursing intervention to implement when a client is having a problem sleeping is to:

a.   check physician orders to see if the client has a sleeping pill ordered.

b.   provide client with a back rub.

c.   determine client's normal bedtime ritual.

d.   reduce environmental noise.

b
Application
Implementation
Physiological:
Pharmacological and
Parenteral Therapies

42-25   A client is being discharged to home with an order for a sedative-hypnotic medication to help him sleep. What information is important to give to the client related to use of the sleep medication?

a.   Use the medication only as a last resort.

b.   The medication may cause drowsiness and a morning hangover.

c.   The medication is addictive and should be used with caution.

d.   The medication causes central nervous system excitability.

d
Application
Implementation
Physiological:
Physiological
Adaptation

43-1   All but one of the following nurses is operating under a common misperception of pain. Which nurse is intervening appropriately and demonstrating a correct understanding of pain?

     a.   Nurse A believes that clients in pain are likely to become addicted, so he advises them to wait as long as possible before requesting prn narcotics.

     b.   A client who is in early labor is crying out, restless, and complaining of pain. Palpating only mild contractions, Nurse B thinks, "She can't be having that much pain so early in labor—not with those mild contractions."

     c.   When a client complains of pain, Nurse C notes no physiological or behavioral signs of pain, so she concludes that his pain is not severe.

     d.   Nurse D assesses all surgery clients carefully for pain, realizing that even minor surgery clients can experience intense pain.

a
Application
Analysis/Diagnosis
Physiological:
Physiological
Adaptation

43-2   The nurse observes the following cues: a client states he is having pain; he grimaces and winces when the nurse helps him turn in bed; his pulse is 120, respirations 30, and he is perspiring. These are defining characteristics for a NANDA nursing diagnosis of:

     a.   Acute Pain.

     b.   Chronic Pain.

     c.   Altered Comfort.

     d.   Impaired Mobility.

a
Comprehension
Analysis/Diagnosis
Physiological:
Physiological
Adaptation

43-3   A client has her right lower leg amputated following an episode of gangrene. Two days later she is complaining of pain in her right great toe. What kind of pain is she having?

     a.   phantom

     b.   referred

     c.   psychogenic

     d.   intractable

d
Application
Analysis/Diagnosis
Physiological:
Physiological
Adaptation

43-4   On returning from surgery, a client initially refuses to take any medication for her pain, stating that she doesn't need it yet. This suggests that she has a:

     a.   low pain threshold.

     b.   high pain threshold.

     c.   low pain tolerance.

     d.   high pain tolerance.

b Knowledge Physiological: Pharmacological and Parenteral Therapies	43-5	Opioid (narcotic) analgesics work physiologically by binding to opiate receptors and: a. decreasing the level of inflammatory mediators at the site of injury. b. activating endogenous pain suppression in the central nervous system. c. decreasing the release of prostaglandins in the central nervous system. d. decreasing the sensitivity of peripheral nerve endings.
a Knowledge Assessment Physiological: Physiological Adaptation	43-6	A four-year-old client has severe abdominal pain. What is the best way for you to find out the exact location of her pain? a. Have her point to where the pain is. b. Ask her to tell you where the pain is. c. Observe for nonverbal behaviors such as guarding of body parts. d. Solicit her mother's cooperation in locating the pain.
a Application Assessment Physiological: Physiological Adaptation	43-7	A four-year-old client has severe abdominal pain. What is the nurse trying to assess when she asks the client's mother if the client has had any nausea and vomiting with her pain? a. associated symptoms b. coping resources c. effect on activities of daily living d. pain relief measures
b Application Implementation Physiological: Pharmacological and Parenteral Therapies	43-8	A client has just returned to his room following back surgery. During the next 24 hours, what is the most effective timing for administration of his prn pain medication? a. when the client requests it b. on a regular schedule c. after the client exhibits signs of pain d. four hours after returning to his room from surgery
b Application Implementation Physiological: Physiological Adaptation	43-9	A four-year-old client is crying and saying, "It hurts." Which of the following nursing interventions is most appropriate in response to the client's perception of the pain? a. Tell him, "Be brave. Big boys don't cry." b. Hold him to provide comfort c. Teach him about the meaning of his pain d. Tell him, "When you cry, it makes it hurt worse."

a
Knowledge
Assessment
Physiological:
Pharmacological and
Parenteral Therapies

43-10 How do narcotics work to achieve pain relief?

a. They alter pain perception.

b. They increase pain tolerance.

c. They remove the pain stimulus.

d. They block nerve transmission.

c
Application
Evaluation
Physiological:
Pharmacological and
Parenteral Therapies

43-11 As a general rule, which of the following would be most important in evaluating whether a client is having side effects from morphine (narcotic) administration?

a. heart rate

b. blood pressure

c. respiratory rate

d. presence of pain

c
Application
Implementation
Physiological:
Reduction of Risk
Potential

43-12 Two hours after receiving his narcotic analgesic, the client is still complaining of severe leg pain. His pain medication cannot be repeated for another hour. How can the nurse best assist him to deal with pain now?

a. Offer him a magazine to read.

b. Turn the lights down and close the door.

c. Guide him in slow, rhythmic breathing techniques.

d. Ask the physician to increase the dosage of his prn pain medication.

a
Knowledge
Assessment
Physiological:
Physiological
Adaptation

43-13 Adjectives such as gnawing, sharp, and piercing describe what aspect of pain assessment?

a. quality

b. duration

c. intensity

d. location

d
Knowledge
Assessment
Physiological:
Growth and
Development
Through the Life
Span

43-14 In which of the following age groups would you expect to find clients with decreased sensation or perception of pain?

a. infant

b. toddler

c. adolescent

d. older adults

a
Knowledge
Planning
Physiological:
Pharmacological and
Parenteral Therapies

43-15 Aspirin is contraindicated in which of the following clients?

a. a client with a peptic ulcer

b. a client with a fractured leg

c. a client with a migraine headache

d. a client with a rheumatoid arthritis

b
Application
Evaluation
Physiological:
Pharmacological and
Parenteral Therapies

43-16 One hour after receiving his pain medication, the client is able to ambulate in the hall for 20 minutes. This indicates that the dosage of pain medication is:

a. excessive.

b. appropriate.

c. insufficient.

d. incorrect.

b
Comprehension
Assessment
Physiological:
Physiological
Adaptation

43-17 A client is suffering from terminal cancer. His pain is severe and resistant to medication or any of the usual pain relief measures. His pain is best described as:

a. chronic.

b. intractable.

c. psychogenic.

d. somatogenic.

d
Knowledge
Assessment
Physiological:
Physiological
Adaptation

43-18 Which of the following characteristics is usually seen in chronic, rather than acute, pain?

a. restlessness and anxiety

b. dilated pupils

c. increased respiratory rate

d. dry, warm skin

a
Knowledge
Implementation
Physiological:
Pharmacological and
Parenteral Therapies

43-19 The physician has ordered patient-controlled analgesia (PCA) for a client with intractable pain. Which of the following equipment will you need when initiating the PCA therapy?

a. gloves

b. conduction cream or gel

c. bath basin with warm water

d. syringe with 1-1/2 inch needle

c
Knowledge
Physiological:
Pharmacological and
Parenteral Therapies

43-20 In an attempt to control a client's intractable pain, the physician has interrupted his nerve pathways with chemical agents. This form of treatment is called:

a. cutaneous stimulation.

b. acupuncture.

c. nerve block.

d. counterirritant therapy.

b
Application
Implementation
Physiological:
Reduction of Risk
Potential

43-21 The physician has ordered that application of a splint to a client's knee for acute pain management. Which of the following statements about the application of the splint is true?

   a. It ensures that the knee remains in place, and it must be used for a least four hours to be effective.
   b. It holds the joints in their position of function, and it should be removed at least every hour.
   c. It should be secured tightly at the insertion point with an elastic bandage.
   d. It should not limit movement of the joint.

c
Application
Implementation
Physiological:
Pharmacological and
Parenteral Therapies

43-22 A postoperative client tells her nurse that she is in pain. On the pain scale (1 to 10, with 1 being the least), the client reports her pain as an 8. The nurse tells the client that she will provide an injection of Demerol (meperidine hydrochloride) as ordered by the physician. The client states that Demerol has never worked for her and that she needs morphine. What is the most appropriate nursing action?

   a. Tell the client that Demerol is what is ordered and administer the medication.
   b. Convince the client that Demerol will work and administer the medication.
   c. Contact the physician and report the client's concern.
   d. Do not give the medication and provide a back massage.

b
Application
Implementation
Physiological:
Physiological
Adaptation

43-23 A client with chronic pain who was started on a fentanyl citrate skin patch one week ago returns to the clinic for a follow-up visit. The client reports that his pain is much better but that he has become constipated. The nurse should

   a. have the client discontinue the fentanyl citrate.
   b. provide information on fluid intake and dietary measures to promote bowel function.
   c. encourage the daily use of an over-the-counter laxative to promote bowel function.
   d. consult with the physician to order a lower GI x-rays.

43-24 A client is receiving intravenous morphine sulfate for pain management. The nurse goes in to the client's room and finds the client sleeping soundly. She calls the client's name and he does not respond. She notes the respiratory rate is 10 and shallow and the client does not respond to tactile stimulation. What should be her first nursing action?

a. Call the physician.

b. Administer Narcan according to the physician's standing orders.

c. Monitor the client's condition; this is an expected response to intravenous morphine.

d. Stop the intravenous infusion of morphine.

43-25 The nurse has instructed a client with chronic pain to keep a daily pain diary. The rationale for having the client keep such a diary is to:

a. make the client document when she has pain.

b. determine when to provide medication to the client.

c. help the nurse and client to identify pain patterns and causative factors.

d. distract the client so that her pain will be reduced.

Application
Assessment
Physiological:
Physiological
Adaptation

44-1 Which of the following would directly interfere with a client's ability to store and convert carbohydrates?

  a. stomach disease

  b. kidney disease

  c. liver disease

  d. lymphatic system disease

Knowledge
Physiological: Basic
Care and Comfort

44-2 Which of the following can be stored in the body, making daily intake unnecessary?

  a. minerals

  b. water-soluble vitamins

  c. fat-soluble vitamins

  d. fiber

Knowledge
Physiological: Basic
Care and Comfort

44-3 Ingested carbohydrates that are not needed for energy are stored either as glycogen or:

  a. fat.

  b. muscle.

  c. pyruvic acid.

  d. glucose.

Knowledge
Physiological: Basic
Care and Comfort

44-4 Which nutrient provides the major source of energy for the body?

  a. fats

  b. carbohydrates

  c. proteins

  d. vitamins

Comprehension
Physiological: Basic
Care and Comfort

44-5 Which of the following foods contains all the essential amino acids?

  a. eggs

  b. whole wheat cereal

  c. potatoes

  d. dried beans

Application
Assessment
Physiological: Basic
Care and Comfort

44-6 Which of the following persons is most likely to have a negative nitrogen balance?

  a. a healthy man who ingests 60 g of protein per day

  b. a holy man who has been on a water-only fast for two weeks

  c. a healthy pregnant woman

  d. a weightlifter who is adding muscle mass

d
Comprehension
Planning
Physiological: Basic
Care and Comfort

44-7 A client needs to avoid saturated fatty acids. The nurse knows that he can best accomplish this by:

a. using only animal fat.

b. reducing his fat intake to 30% of total calories.

c. avoiding all fats and fatty foods.

d. using fats that are liquid at room temperature.

a
Application
Physiological: Basic
Care and Comfort

44-8 Using the Food Guide Pyramid as a standard, which of the following is an adequate daily intake of the milk-yogurt-cheese group?

a. a glass of milk and 1 serving of cheese

b. a glass of milk

c. 1/2 cup of unflavored yogurt

d. 1/2 cup of yogurt and 1 egg

d
Knowledge
Planning
Physiological:
Growth and
Development
Through the Life
Span

44-9 The elderly adult needs a daily intake of at least _____ mg calcium to prevent bone loss.

a. 60

b. 160

c. 600

d. 800

c
Application
Implementation
Physiological: Basic
Care and Comfort

44-10 What is the most important action a nurse can take in promoting good nutrition for a hospitalized 89-year-old Hispanic client?

a. Explain that tamales contain meat and spices that are not good for her.

b. Request that the dietitian add peppers and tortillas to her menu.

c. Find out what the client likes to eat and try to include that in her diet.

d. Teach her the foods suggested by the Food Guide Pyramid.

a
Knowledge
Assessment
Promotion:
Prevention and Early
Detection of Disease

44-11 Which of the following assessments is used to determine whether a person's weight is appropriate to his or her height?

a. body mass index

b. serum albumin

c. skinfold measurements

d. total daily calorie consumption

b
Application
Assessment
Physiological: Basic
Care and Comfort

44-12 Which of the following clients may be exhibiting signs of poor nutritional status?

a. a client whose hair is shiny, and neither dry nor oily

b. a client whose skin is dry and rough with a few bruises

c. a client whose tongue and mucous membranes are pink and moist

d. a client whose body mass index is 26

44-13   Which of the following is the best indicator of iron deficiency?

a.   low hemoglobin level

b.   low serum albumin

c.   decreased creatinine excretion

d.   decreased total lymphocyte count

44-14   A 42-year-old Mexican-American client refuses to eat the hospital-prepared foods and eats only the flour tortillas, beans, and rice brought in by her family. The nurse's first action should be to:

a.   determine whether the client's diet meets her daily nutritional requirements.

b.   find out how to add meat to the client's diet for necessary protein intake.

c.   tell the client that the hospital prepares a balanced meal, and it would be better for her to eat what is on her tray.

d.   explain to the client how she can choose items of preference from the hospital menu.

44-15   Which of the following menus is acceptable for a client on a clear liquid diet?

a.   milk, coffee, and apple juice

b.   tea, cola, and gelatin

c.   water, tea, coffee, and ice cream

d.   milk, gelatin, and cola

44-16   A client has just returned to the unit after undergoing eye surgery. He has bandages on both eyes. When his lunch tray is delivered, the best intervention for the nurse would be to:

a.   open all containers and leave, letting him be as independent as possible.

b.   feed him, allowing sufficient time for tasting, chewing, and swallowing.

c.   cut his meat into bite-size pieces and tell him the position of the food according to the hours of a clock.

d.   keep him on a liquid diet until the bandages are removed.

44-17   Which of the following community nutritional services would be appropriate to recommend to a 45-year-old, divorced, unemployed mother of three children?

a.   Title III meals

b.   a food stamp program

c.   Meals on Wheels

d.   the Nutrition Program for Older Americans

b
Knowledge
Analysis/Diagnosis
Pharmacological and
Parenteral Therapies

44-18   Diarrhea is a common problem associated with tube feedings. Which of the following is a cause of diarrhea in clients on tube feedings?

a. improper tube placement

b. a formula with a high osmolality

c. improper positioning of the client during the feeding

d. inadequate fluid intake

a
Comprehension
Physiological:
Pharmacological and
Parenteral Therapies

44-19   Which of the following is true of a gastrostomy feeding tube?

a. It allows the client greater mobility and enables self-feeding.

b. It is inserted through one of the nostrils, down the esophagus, and into the stomach.

c. It enters a surgical opening through the small intestine.

d. It must be used in conjunction with a feeding pump.

b
Application
Planning
Health Promotion:
Prevention and Early
Detection of Disease

44-20   A mother brings her 14-year-old son into the clinic for his annual sports physical exam. When the clinic nurse asks the mother if she has any concerns, she responds that she thinks her son is eating too much and will become fat like her. The nurse takes her son's height and weight and determines that his weight within normal limits. What should be the focus of the nutrition education provided to the mother?

a. showing the mother how to calculate her son's caloric needs

b. discussing nutritional needs during periods of growth

c. prevention of obesity in adolescents

d. prevention of food fads which occur during adolescence

c
Comprehension
Assessment
Physiological:
Reduction of Risk
Potential

44-21   At an immunization clinic, the nurse notices that a very young infant is in her car seat with a bottle propped in her mouth. The nurse identifies that this type of feeding can result in:

a. overfeeding.

b. introduction of too much air into the infant's abdomen.

c. aspiration.

d. sudden infant death syndrome.

Application
Evaluation
Physiological:
Pharmacological and
Parenteral Therapies

44-22 A client who is receiving parenteral feedings will be going home. The nurse has just finished providing the client information on the care of the access device. The nurse knows the client understands the information when he says:

a. "It is important to wash my hands after I change the dressing and to make sure no one touches the site."

b. "It is important not to move when the bag is attached so it will go in properly."

c. "It is important that I look at the device site daily, take my temperature, and call if I think there is a problem."

d. "It is alright to use the same dressing two days in a row."

Application
Planning
Physiological: Basic
Care and Comfort

44-23 The discharge planning nurse is reviewing the medical record of a client who was admitted for gall bladder surgery and is being discharged. The admission nursing assessment indicates the client is more than 20% below her ideal weight, with poor short-term memory. How can the discharge nurse help the client meet her nutritional needs at home?

a. Discuss the client's nutritional needs and recommend follow-up visits to the health care provider.

b. Provide written nutritional information, and make a recommendation for referral to Meals on Wheels.

c. Suggest to the family that it is time to seek an alternative living situation for the client.

d. Provide a referral to adult protective services to ensure the client's living situation is healthy.

Application
Implementation
Physiological: Basic
Care and Comfort

44-24 What should a nurse do to stimulate the appetite of a client who is not eating well?

a. Have the family bring large, attractive portions of food to provide to the client.

b. Provide food that the client likes and relieve symptoms of illness.

c. Provide treatments before meal time so the client doesn't have to think about them while eating.

d. Provide meals after the client has been active because activity increases appetite.

44-25   In order to aspirate gastric contents from a small-bore feeding tube, the nurse knows that it may be necessary to:

a.   use a smaller syringe (10 cc) because it will decrease the possibility of collapsing the tube.

b.   use a larger syringe (30 cc) because it will create less negative pressure.

c.   use a suction machine and set it to continuous suction.

d.   use a smaller syringe (10 cc) because it will create positive pressure.

a
Knowledge
Physiological: Basic
Care and Comfort

45-1 A function of mucus in the large intestine is to:

    a. protect the intestinal wall from fecal acids and bacterial activity.

    b. control the amount of flatus produced by carbohydrate digestion.

    c. promote movement of the chyme within the haustra.

    d. stimulate the intrinsic defecation reflex.

d
Application
Implementation
Physiological: Basic
Care and Comfort

45-2 An 80-year-old client is worried because she has not had a bowel movement every day. Which statement by her nurse reflects the best understanding of defecation patterns?

    a. "A bowel movement each day is the normal pattern for most people. We will ask for a laxative order for you."

    b. "You shouldn't worry until you have gone at least three days without a bowel movement."

    c. "You need to eat more fiber to stimulate daily bowel movements. Can I get you some prunes?"

    d. "The number of bowel movements per week varies greatly. It can be quite normal to have only two or three bowel movements per week."

a
Comprehension
Assessment
Physiological:
Growth and
Development
Through the Life
Span

45-3 What physiological changes of aging predispose elderly clients to constipation?

    a. loss of tonus of the smooth muscle of the colon

    b. decreased control of anal sphincter muscles

    c. inhibition of the parasympathetic defecation reflex

    d. inability to absorb fluid from the chyme in the colon

b
Knowledge
Analysis/Diagnosis
Physiological: Basic
Care and Comfort

45-4 Which of the following contributes to constipation?

    a. high-fiber diets

    b. overuse and prolonged use of laxatives

    c. excessive exercise

    d. having a regular time each day for defecation

b
Knowledge
Analysis/Diagnosis
Physiological:
Physiological
Adaptation

45-5 The temporary cessation of intestinal movement following surgical manipulation of the intestines is termed:

    a. atony.

    b. paralytic ileus.

    c. impaction.

    d. flatulence.

d Knowledge Physiological: Pharmacological and Parenteral Therapies	45-6	An example of a drug that causes constipation by acting on the central nervous system to slow motility of the colon is: a. Surfak. b. Metamucil. c. Colace. d. morphine.
c Comprehension Analysis/Diagnosis Physiological: Physiological Adaptation	45-7	Which of the following findings is indicative of a fecal impaction? a. loss of desire to defecate b. alternating patterns of normal stool and diarrhea c. constipation with liquid fecal seepage d. absence of stool upon digital rectal exam
a Knowledge Planning Physiological: Basic Care and Comfort	45-8	Which of the following promotes normal defecation? a. providing privacy for defecation b. limiting the client's fluid intake c. having the client use laxatives d. ignoring the duodenocolic reflex
a Knowledge Assessment Physiological: Physiological Adaptation	45-9	The most serious problem arising from severe diarrhea is the potential for: a. fluid and electrolyte loss. b. spasmodic abdominal cramps. c. irritation of the anal region. d. loss of intestinal mucus.
a Knowledge Assessment Physiological: Physiological Adaptation	45-10	What is the usual color of the stools of a client experiencing upper GI tract bleeding? a. black b. clay-colored c. bright red d. greenish
d Knowledge Assessment Physiological: Reduction of Risk Potential	45-11	The guaiac test is one of several bedside procedures to detect the presence of _____ in a stool specimen. a. bile b. helminth infestations c. microorganisms d. blood

b
Knowledge
Assessment
Safety: Safety and
Infection Control

45-12 When collecting a stool specimen from a bedpan, the nurse should:

a. wear sterile gloves and use a sterile specimen cup.

b. be careful not to contaminate the outside of the specimen container with feces.

c. take the specimen to the laboratory at the end of the shift.

d. wearing gloves, remove the specimen from the pan with a paper towel and transfer it to the specimen cup.

a
Application
Analysis/Diagnosis
Physiological: Basic
Care and Comfort

45-13 A 24-year-old client with a fractured femur is confined to bed and is in traction. He states he feels fullness in his rectum and wants to move his bowels, but cannot. His last BM was four days ago. On auscultation, the nurse notes decreased bowel sounds. Which of the following is an appropriate nursing diagnosis for the client?

a. Constipation related to inadequate physical activity

b. Constipation related to inadequate intake of fluids and fiber

c. Perceived Constipation related to knowledge deficit about normal processes

d. Impaired Skin Integrity related to immobility

c
Application
Planning
Physiological: Basic
Care and Comfort

45-14 Which of the following is the most appropriate outcome criterion for a client with constipation?

a. The client will remain free of perianal irritation and odor.

b. The client will participate actively in a bowel training program.

c. The client will consume a well-balanced diet that includes fiber and 8 to 10 glasses of fluid daily.

d. The client will be free of flatulence.

d
Comprehension
Assessment
Physiological:
Reduction of Risk
Potential

45-15 The nurse should observe the client for the side effect of water intoxication after administering which type of enema?

a. oil

b. soap

c. hypertonic

d. hypotonic

b
Knowledge
Physiological: Basic
Care and Comfort

45-16 Which of the following is considered to be a slow-acting type of cathartic?

a. lubricants

b. wetting agents

c. chemical stimulants

d. saline

c
Knowledge
Implementation
Physiological: Basic
Care and Comfort

45-17 A carminative enema acts by:

a. distending the intestine with a large volume of fluid.

b. lubricating the rectum and anal canal to make evacuation easier.

c. distending the rectum and colon with gas released from the enema solution.

d. alternating flow of fluid into and out of the large intestine.

b
Knowledge
Implementation
Physiological: Basic
Care and Comfort

45-18 A return flow enema, also known as a colonic irrigation, is used to:

a. soften feces.

b. expel flatus.

c. administer medications.

d. clean the rectum of fecal contents.

d
Application
Implementation
Physiological: Basic
Care and Comfort

45-19 A client with a new ileostomy asks the nurse when his fecal output will become "regulated." Which response by the nurse demonstrates correct understanding of ileostomy drainage?

a. "Your ileostomy output will become regulated as the drainage becomes more solid."

b. "Your ileostomy output will be regulated when you begin to irrigate it daily."

c. "You will be able to regulate the ileostomy output by following a special diet."

d. "Your ileostomy will produce liquid drainage continuously; regulation is not possible."

a
Application
Planning
Physiological:
Physiological
Adaptation

45-20 When assessing a client's colostomy stoma, the nurse notes that it is dark blue in color. The nurse should:

a. notify the physician immediately.

b. apply an antibiotic powder to the stoma surface.

c. remove the old Karaya wafer and apply a new one to the stoma area.

d. use only hypoallergenic adhesive on the ostomy appliance.

d
Knowledge
Implementation
Physiological: Basic
Care and Comfort

45-21 Which of the following is a correct part of the procedure for changing of bowel diversion ostomy appliance?

a. Schedule the ostomy change for 30 to 45 minutes before meal time.

b. Don sterile gloves before removing the ostomy pouch.

c. Peel the bag off quickly to decrease the amount of pain.

d. Empty the pouch into a bedpan before removing the ostomy appliance.

45-22 A mother comes to the well child clinic with her one-month-old infant. She tells the nurse that she is going to have to stop breastfeeding because her baby's stools are yellow. What is the nurse's best response?

    a. "It is normal for your breastfed infant to have yellow stools. Is there any other reason you feel you should quit breastfeeding?"

    b. "You feel that because your baby's stools are yellow you are not providing the right kind of feeding for her?"

    c. "You're right. Let's discuss this problem with the doctor."

    d. "You really don't need to worry. It is normal for the baby's stools to be that color."

45-23 A client has been put on a low-residue diet. To prevent constipation, it is important that the nurse instruct the client to:

    a. use an over-the-counter laxative every other day.

    b. increase his daily fluid intake.

    c. increase the amount rice he eats daily.

    d. decrease his physical activity.

45-24 What is the first nursing action in initiating a bowel training program for a client?

    a. increase the client's fluid intake

    b. administer a suppository

    c. assess the client's usual bowel habits

    d. increase the fiber in the client's diet

45-25 What is a nursing priority for a client using a rectal pouch?

    a. maintaining normal fluid balance

    b. promoting adequate nutrition

    c. regular assessment of the perianal skin

    d. positioning for defecation

45-26 A nurse encounters resistance at the internal sphincter during insertion of an enema tube into the client. What is the next nursing action?

    a. Raise the height of the container holding the solution to increase the pressure.

    b. Withdraw the tube right away, and report resistance to the charge nurse.

    c. Instruct the client to take a deep breath, and run a small amount of fluid through the tube.

    d. Withdraw the tube and then re-insert.

a
Knowledge
Assessment
Physiological: Basic
Care and Comfort

46-1   Which of the following is a characteristic of normal urine?

    a.   It appears transparent.

    b.   It has a musty odor.

    c.   It contains mucous.

    d.   It is dark amber in color.

a
Knowledge
Assessment
Physiological:
Physiological
Adaptation

46-2   Which of the following, if found in the urine, is a sign of glomerular injury?

    a.   protein

    b.   ketone bodies

    c.   glucose

    d.   microorganisms

b
Knowledge
Physiological: Basic
Care and Comfort

46-3   At a cellular level, the basic unit of functioning of the renal system is the:

    a.   neuron.

    b.   nephron.

    c.   glomerulus.

    d.   bladder.

b
Comprehension
Assessment
Physiological:
Reduction of Risk
Potential

46-4   A client delivered her first child, a four-pound male, six hours ago. She suffered post-delivery complications and was transferred to the obstetric intensive care unit in critical but stable condition. You would notify her obstetrician if her urinary output falls below:

    a.   15 cc per hour.

    b.   30 cc per hour.

    c.   60 cc per hour.

    d.   100 cc per hour.

b
Knowledge
Assessment
Physiological:
Physiological
Adaptation

46-5   The production of scant amounts of urine, such as 100 to 500 ml per day, is referred to as:

    a.   anuria.

    b.   oliguria.

    c.   dysuria.

    d.   retention.

d
Knowledge
Assessment
Physiological:
Reduction of Risk
Potential

46-6   A hydrometer is used to measure:

a.   pH of urine.

b.   hourly urine amounts.

c.   temperature of urine at voiding.

d.   specific gravity of urine.

c
Application
Assessment
Physiological:
Physiological
Adaptation

46-7   A client tells the nurse, "The need to urinate comes on me all of a sudden, and it feels as though I have to go immediately—that I can't wait." The nurse would chart that the client is experiencing:

a.   urinary frequency.

b.   enuresis.

c.   urinary urgency.

d.   dysuria.

b
Comprehension
Analysis/Diagnosis
Physiological:
Physiological
Adaptation

46-8   A client feels discomfort in his pubic area. He tells the nurse he has been voiding "only a little bit, about every half hour." These are clinical signs of:

a.   functional incontinence.

b.   retention.

c.   nocturia.

d.   stress incontinence.

a
Knowledge
Assessment
Physiological:
Reduction of Risk
Potential

46-9   An advantage of the ileal conduit over ureterostomies is that with an ileal conduit there is:

a.   less chance of an ascending kidney infection.

b.   more control over urinary elimination.

c.   a smaller stoma, which is more easily fitted to an appliance.

d.   no need for an external collection device.

b
Comprehension
Analysis/Diagnosis
Physiological:
Reduction of Risk
Potential

46-10   Which of the following clients should be observed for development of urinary retention?

a.   a client who is taking aspirin four times a day for arthritis

b.   a client who is taking an antihistamine preparation for allergies

c.   a client who is drinking one or two alcoholic beverages each day

d.   a client who is taking furosemide (a diuretic)

c
Application
Analysis/Diagnosis
Physiological:
Physiological
Adaptation

46-11   A client suffered a spinal cord injury in a motorcycle accident nine months ago. He has no awareness of bladder filling, urge to void, or feelings of bladder fullness. He reports loss of urine at fairly frequent intervals—about every two hours. Which of the following is a correct nursing diagnosis for Tim?

a.   Functional Incontinence related to spinal cord injury

b.   Urinary Retention related to paralysis

c.   Risk for Impaired Skin Integrity related to incontinence

d.   Impaired Skin Integrity related to incontinence

b
Application
Analysis/Diagnosis
Physiological:
Physiological
Adaptation

46-12   A client suffered a spinal cord injury in a motorcycle accident nine months ago. He has no awareness of bladder filling, urge to void, or feelings of bladder fullness. He reports loss of urine at fairly frequent intervals—about every two hours. What type of incontinence is he most likely experiencing?

a.   functional incontinence

b.   reflex incontinence

c.   stress incontinence

d.   urge incontinence

a
Comprehension
Implementation
Physiological: Basic
Care and Comfort

46-13   A client has an indwelling catheter. Many procedures involving the organs of elimination are embarrassing to the client. Therefore, when performing catheter care, it is most important for you to:

a.   provide privacy and use proper draping procedures.

b.   ask the client to tell you why he is embarrassed.

c.   work quickly in order to decrease the client's discomfort.

c.   tell the client this is routine care and not to be embarrassed.

c
Comprehension
Implementation
Physiological:
Reduction of Risk
Potential

46-14   You are securing a retention catheter by taping it to the client's leg. She asks why it is necessary. What is your best response?

a.   "It is important for preventing urinary leakage around the catheter."

b.   "It is important for preventing the catheter from slipping out of your bladder."

c.   "It is important for preventing trauma to your external urethral sphincter."

d.   "It is important for preventing urinary tract infection."

c
Comprehension
Implementation
Physiological:
Reduction of Risk
Potential

46-15 A client is scheduled for a chest x-ray today. She is ambulatory but still has her indwelling catheter. What instructions should you give to the x-ray technician who accompanies the client to the radiology department?

a. The client may feel abdominal pressure while she is walking about.

b. He should disconnect the drainage bag before leaving the client's room.

c. The drainage bag should be kept below the waist level at all times.

d. The drainage bag should be placed on the x-ray table beside the client during the procedure.

b
Knowledge
Assessment
Physiological:
Reduction of Risk
Potential

46-16 Which of the following is a purpose of urinary catheterization?

a. preventing urinary tract infection

b. assessing the amount of residual urine

c. keeping a client's bed dry

d. obtaining a specimen to examine for protein

c
Knowledge
Implementation
Physiological: Basic
Care and Comfort

46-17 When cleansing the female genitalia immediately prior to catheterization, the correct technique includes:

a. cleansing from front to back without separating the labia.

b. cleansing the perineum with alcohol.

c. separating the labia and cleansing from back to front.

d. separating the labia and cleansing from front to back.

d
Knowledge
Implementation
Physiological:
Reduction of Risk
Potential

46-18 When preparing to insert a straight catheter, as in catheterizing for residual, you will need:

a. a syringe (prefilled with water).

b. nonallergenic tape.

c. a urinary drainage bag.

d. lubricant.

c
Comprehension
Implementation
Physiological:
Reduction of Risk
Potential

46-19 A client has an indwelling catheter. Which of the following interventions should be instituted to help prevent a catheter-associated urine infection?

a. Encourage her to limit fluids to less than 1000 cc per day.

b. Change her catheter every 7 to 10 days.

c. Maintain a closed drainage system.

d. Cleanse her urinary meatus daily with iodine.

d
Knowledge
Implementation
Physiological:
Reduction of Risk
Potential

46-20 Which of the following should be included in teaching a female client health promotion measures regarding urinary elimination?

    a. "If burning accompanies voiding or if the urine becomes cloudy, increase your fluid intake and drink cranberry juice."

    b. "After urination, wipe from the anus toward the urinary meatus."

    c. "To strengthen sphincter muscles, do not void when you first feel the urge; wait as long as you can."

    d. "Empty the bladder at each voiding."

a
Application
Assessment
Physiological:
Reduction of Risk
Potential

46-21 A client's history indicates that she a problem with urination, so the nurse assesses the client's skin for color, texture, tissue turgor, and edema. What is the rationale for these added assessments?

    a. problems with urinary elimination may affect how the body eliminates wastes

    b. the assessments help to obtain information on the client's hydration status

    c. to validate the urinary problem identified by the client

    d. the skin is the largest organ and should always be assessed

a
Comprehension
Assessment
Physiological:
Reduction of Risk
Potential

46-22 A client is admitted to the medical unit with a medical diagnosis of dehydration. What should the nurse expect the client's urine specific gravity to be?

    a. normal

    b. higher than normal

    c. lower than normal

    d. related to the urinary pH

b
Application
Planning
Physiological:
Reduction of Risk
Potential

46-23 A client with a history of renal calculi should be instructed to:

    a. strain all urine.

    b. increase fluid intake to maintain dilute urine.

    c. avoid urinating frequently.

    d. drink a lot of milk.

b
Application
Implementation
Physiological:
Reduction of Risk
Potential

46-24　A client is being discharged to home with a urinary retention catheter. Part of the discharge instructions included encouraging the client to eat whole grains, cranberries, plums, prunes, and to limit fruit, vegetables, and milk products. What is the purpose of these instructions?

a. to prevent urinary tract infections by keeping the urine pH above 7.5

b. to prevent urinary tract infections by keeping the urine pH below 7.5

c. to provide general information on nutritional requirements

d. to promote optimal functioning of the kidneys by reducing the protein in the diet

a
Application
Planning
Physiological: Basic
Care and Comfort

46-25　To promote normal urinary elimination for a client confined to bed the nurse should:

a. warm the bed pan and help the client to simulate normal voiding position.

b. apply cold water over the perineum.

c. perform Crede's maneuver.

d. show client how to inhibit the urge to void.

a
Knowledge
Physiological:
Physiological
Adaptation

47-1   Normal breathing depends partly upon the ability of lung tissue to stretch and recoil. Another important factor is:

    a.   negative intrapleural pressure.

    b.   positive intrapleural pressure.

    c.   absence of intrapulmonic pressure.

    d.   equal intrapleural and intrapulmonic pressures.

a
Knowledge
Assessment
Physiological:
Physiological
Adaptation

47-2   The normal volume of air inspired and expired is called:

    a.   tidal volume.

    b.   inspiratory reserve volume.

    c   total lung capacity.

    d.   vital capacity.

a
Knowledge
Assessment
Physiological:
Physiological
Adaptation

47-3   The respiratory control center is located in the:

    a.   medulla and pons.

    b.   hypothalamus.

    c.   cerebellum.

    d.   pituitary.

d
Application
Analysis/Diagnosis
Physiological:
Physiological
Adaptation

47-4   Which of the following clients is at most immediate risk for being unable to maintain clear air passages?

    a.   a client who has a low hemoglobin level

    b.   a client who gets very little exercise

    c.   a client whose chemoreceptors have become insensitive to carbon dioxide

    d.   a client whose vagus nerve has been damaged

a
Application
Analysis/Diagnosis
Physiological:
Reduction of Risk
Potential

47-5   Which of the following clients should be watched most closely for a problem with the transport of oxygen from the lungs to the tissues?

    a.   a client who has anemia

    b.   a client who has an infection

    c.   a client who has a broken rib

    d.   a client who has a tumor of the medulla

b
Knowledge
Assessment
Physiological:
Physiological
Adaptation

47-6   A normal respiratory rate for the average adult is:

    a.   8 to 14 per minute.

    b.   12 to 20 per minute.

    c.   20 to 40 per minute.

    d.   30 to 80 per minute.

c
Comprehension
Assessment
Physiological:
Physiological
Adaptation

47-7 A client has dyspnea when lying down and must assume an upright or sitting position in order to breathe more comfortably and effectively. The nurse should chart this condition as:

a. dyspnea.
b. hyperpnea.
c. orthopnea.
d. acapnea.

b
Knowledge
Assessment
Physiological:
Physiological
Adaptation

47-8 The term that refers specifically to reduced oxygen in the blood is:

a. hypoxia.
b. hypoxemia.
c. cyanosis.
d. eupnea.

a
Application
Analysis/Diagnosis
Physiological:
Physiological
Adaptation

47-9 A 72-year-old client with chronic obstructive pulmonary disease lived for many years in San Francisco, California (near sea level). When he moved to Denver, Colorado (one mile above sea level), he experienced exacerbation of his disease and was admitted to the emergency room for treatment. A logical explanation is that the client is reacting to:

a. the lower oxygen and barometric pressure in Denver.
b. anxiety related to crowded living conditions in the city.
c. the higher concentration of oxygen found at high altitudes.
d. the atmospheric differences in the heavy, cold air in Denver and the warmer air in San Francisco.

b
Application
Analysis/Diagnosis
Physiological:
Physiological
Adaptation

47-10 The intensive care nurse has had to suction the tracheostomy tube of a 70-year-old client with emphysema every hour for thick, tenacious secretions. His respiratory rate is 34 per minute. On auscultation of his lungs, the nurse notes crackles, wheezes, and coarse sounds over the bronchi. The client seems very tired and has only a weak cough. Based on this data, the most appropriate nursing diagnosis for this client is:

a. Ineffective Breathing Pattern related to fatigue and pain.
b. Ineffective Airway Clearance related to excessive, thick tracheobronchial secretions.
c. Sleep Pattern Disturbance related to dyspnea and fatigue.
d. Powerlessness related to inability to maintain independence associated with COPD.

a
Application
Planning
Physiological:
Physiological
Adaptation

47-11 For a client with a nursing diagnosis of Ineffective Airway related to tracheobronchial obstruction, an essential outcome criteria to include in the care plan is:

a clear breath sounds bilaterally.

b. all pulses palpable and strong.

c. normal arterial blood gases.

d. performs activities of daily living without shortness of breath.

b
Application
Planning
Physiological:
Physiological
Adaptation

47-12 A client has a nursing diagnosis of Ineffective Airway Clearance related to inadequate chest excursion and poor cough effort secondary to pain from chest trauma. What is an appropriate nursing order to help him achieve the outcome of a patent airway?

a. Provide uninterrupted periods of sleep.

b. Encourage and assist with frequent position changes.

c. Assess for cyanosis and clubbing of the fingers.

d. Teach the rationale for his clear liquid diet.

d
Application
Evaluation
Physiological:
Physiological
Adaptation

47-13 A client has a nursing diagnosis of Ineffective Airway Clearance related to inadequate chest excursion and poor cough effort related to pain secondary to trauma. To best evaluate whether he has achieved the outcome of a patent airway, the nurse should:

a. examine his fingers for cyanosis and clubbing.

b. assess his level of anxiety.

c. measure his respiratory excursion.

d. auscultate his lungs.

d
Knowledge
Assessment
Physiological:
Physiological
Adaptation

47-14 To prepare a client for an outpatient chest x-ray, the clinic nurse should:

a. assure that a consent form has been signed.

b. explain that it will detect blood flow abnormalities.

c. spray a local anesthetic in her throat.

d. have her remove her jewelry and clothing from the waist up.

b
Knowledge
Assessment
Safety: Safety and
Infection Control

47-15 Which of the following is a sterile procedure?

a. pulmonary function tests

b. bronchoscopy

c. chest x-ray

d. lung scan

c
Comprehension
Planning
Physiological:
Reduction of Risk
Potential

47-16 Which intervention strengthens respiratory and abdominal muscles and promotes gaseous exchange by inflating the lungs?

a. IPPB treatments

b. coughing exercises

c. breathing exercises

d. percussion and vibration

a
Knowledge
Implementation
Physiological:
Physiological
Adaptation

47-17 When instructing a client about pursed-lip breathing, the nurse should tell the client to inhale:

a. through the nose and exhale through pursed lips.

b. through the mouth and exhale through pursed lips.

c. and exhale through pursed lips.

d. through pursed lips and exhale through the nose.

c
Application
Evaluation
Physiological:
Physiological
Adaptation

47-18 Which of the following would indicate that a client with a nursing diagnosis of Ineffective Breathing Pattern is achieving the goal of establishing a normal, effective respiratory pattern?

a. He has an effective cough effort.

b. His intake is 2000 mL/day of fluids.

c. He breathes without use of accessory muscles.

d. His respiratory rate of 30 to 40 per minute.

d
Application
Assessment
Physiological:
Reduction of Risk
Potential

47-19 When a client is receiving oxygen therapy through a nasal cannula delivery system, the nursing care must include:

a. removing the cannula when the client is eating or drinking.

b. assuring that the rebreather bag does not totally deflate.

c. checking the color code on the cannula to determine the precise oxygen concentration.

d. inspecting the nares for encrustation and irritation.

b
Comprehension
Implementation
Physiological:
Reduction of Risk
Potential

47-20 Which of the following is an appropriate safety precaution to observe with the use of oxygen therapy?

a. Use woolen or synthetic blankets on the bed.

b. Be sure that electric monitoring equipment is grounded.

c. Keep a fire extinguisher by the bedside.

d. Clean the equipment and tubing with alcohol daily.

47-21 When suctioning a client with a tracheostomy, the purpose of using an unsterile glove is to:

    a. prevent the transmission of microorganisms to the nurse.

    b. prevent the transmission of microorganisms to the client.

    c. attach the catheter to suction.

    d. keep the suction catheter clean.

47-22 How long can the brain be deprived of oxygen without suffering extensive and permanent damage?

    a. 30 to 60 seconds

    b. 1 to 3 minutes

    c. 4 to 6 minutes

    d. 8 to 10 minutes

47-23 A client has a very shallow breathing pattern that is interrupted by periods of apnea. The nurse should chart this as:

    a. Cheyne-Stokes respirations.

    b. Kussmaul's respirations.

    c. Biot's breathing.

    d. Apneustic breathing.

47-24 The proper position for a chest tube drainage system is:

    a. at the level of the client's right atrium.

    b. below the level of the client's chest.

    c. just above the level of the client's chest.

    d. at the level of the client's diaphragm.

47-25 During the nursing assessment of a client the nurse notes the anteroposterior diameter of the chest is two times smaller that its transverse diameter. The nurse documents this finding as a:

    a. pigeon chest.

    b. funnel chest.

    c. barrel chest.

    d. pectus carinatum.

47-26 The nurse needs to collect a sputum specimen from a client for acid-fast bacillus. The best time to collect this specimen is:

    a. after breakfast in which the client has had milk.

    b. in the afternoon.

    c. at bed time.

    d. in the morning after the client awakens.

c
Application
Planning
Physiological:
Reduction of Risk
Potential

47-27 What is a nursing intervention to maintain normal respiratory function for a client who is receiving narcotics for pain management?

a. Position legs in elevated position.

b. Maintain the head of bed in semi-Fowler's position.

c. Make frequent position changes.

d. Reduce fluid intake.

b
Application
Planning
Physiological:
Reduction of Risk
Potential

47-28 What equipment should a nurse ensure is at the bedside of a client with a chest tube?

a. crash cart

b. rubber-tipped clamps and sterile occlusive dressing

c. endotracheal tube and suction equipment

d. partial rebreather oxygen mask

c
Application
Planning
Physiological:
Physiological
Adaptation

47-29 A goal of ensuring adequate tissue perfusion has been established for a client with anemia. What would be a desired outcome for this goal?

a. Has symmetrical chest expansion.

b. Uses pursed-lip breathing.

c. Has brisk capillary refill.

d. Has activity intolerance.

a
Application
Implementation
Promotion:
Prevention and Early
Detection of Disease

47-30 The home health nurse has developed a teaching guide for her client that focuses on the importance of regular physical activity with gradually increasing activity levels. This teaching guide specifically promotes:

a. cardiac output and tissue perfusion.

b. renal perfusion and formation of urine.

c. oxygen-carrying capacity of white blood cells.

d. effective breathing and airway clearance.

a
Application
Assessment
Physiological:
Physiological
Adaptation

48-1   Which of the following clients is most at risk for fluid imbalance?

    a.   an infant with diarrhea

    b.   an adolescent mowing the lawn on a hot day

    c.   a healthy 70-year-old man with a fractured wrist

    d.   a middle-aged woman who is vomiting

a
Knowledge
Physiological:
Physiological
Adaptation

48-2   What are the principal ions found in the extracellular fluids?

    a.   sodium and chloride

    b.   potassium and phosphate

    c.   sodium and potassium

    d.   potassium and protein

b
Knowledge
Physiological:
Physiological
Adaptation

48-3   Fluids in the interstitial spaces are called:

    a.   intracellular fluids.

    b.   extracellular fluids.

    c.   electrolytes.

    d.   intravascular fluids.

c
Knowledge
Physiological:
Physiological
Adaptation

48-4   The movement of particles from an area of high solute concentration to an area of lower solute concentration is called:

    a.   filtration.

    b.   hydrostatic pressure.

    c.   diffusion.

    d.   osmosis.

d
Knowledge
Analysis/Diagnosis
Physiological:
Physiological
Adaptation

48-5   Which of the following stimulates the thirst center in the hypothalamus?

    a.   high blood pressure

    b.   decreased release of angiotensin II

    c.   release of antidiuretic hormone from the pituitary gland

    d.   decrease in blood volume

c
Knowledge
Planning
Physiological:
Pharmacological and
Parenteral Therapies

48-6   Intravenous solutions are usually:

    a.   hypertonic.

    b.   hypotonic.

    c.   isotonic.

    d.   hyperosmotic.

c
Knowledge
Assessment
Physiological:
Reduction of Risk
Potential

48-7   Blood chemistry is slightly alkaline but is considered physiologically neutral, with a normal pH of:

a. 7.2.

b. 7.3.

c. 7.4.

d. 7.5.

a
Comprehension
Assessment
Promotion:
Prevention and Early
Detection of Disease

48-8   When individuals are in a well or healthy state, their fluid output should be:

a. approximately the same as their fluid intake.

b. correlated very little with their fluid intake.

c. higher than their fluid intake.

d. lower than their fluid intake.

a
Application
Planning
Physiological:
Physiological
Adaptation

48-9   A client is experiencing stress because the reason for her present illness is unknown. She is anxious about the diagnostic testing she is about to undergo. The nurse notices a decrease in the client's urine output and interprets this as an expected response to her stress. The nurse's intervention should be to:

a. not intervene at this time.

b. increase the amount of fluids the client is receiving.

c. notify the physician and request an order for a diuretic.

d. decrease the client's fluid intake in order to maintain a balance.

c
Comprehension
Assessment
Physiological:
Physiological
Adaptation

48-10   For an individual experiencing an intracellular fluid deficit, an appropriate nursing intervention would be to:

a. restrict fluids.

b. administer diuretics as ordered.

c. observe for an increase in temperature.

d. observe for dyspnea and shortness of breath.

c
Knowledge
Physiological:
Physiological
Adaptation

48-11   Plasma proteins help contain blood within the blood vessels by exerting:

a. filtration pressure.

b. hydrostatic pressure.

c. colloid osmotic pressure.

d. diffusion pressure.

b
Comprehension
Analysis/Diagnosis
Physiological:
Physiological
Adaptation

48-12 A client is experiencing tingling of her fingers and toes, muscle cramps, and numbness of her extremities. She may be exhibiting symptoms of:

a. sodium excess.

b. calcium deficit.

c. magnesium excess.

d. chloride deficit.

a
Comprehension
Assessment
Physiological:
Physiological
Adaptation

48-13 For a client with severe diarrhea, the nurse must be alert for the development of the physiological complication of:

a. metabolic acidosis.

b. metabolic alkalosis.

c. respiratory acidosis.

d. respiratory alkalosis.

d
Comprehension
Planning
Physiological:
Physiological
Adaptation

48-14 A client reports that she takes large amounts of antacids for relief of her "acid indigestion." In client teaching, the nurse should explain to the client that this practice may cause:

a. respiratory alkalosis with numbness and dizziness.

b. respiratory acidosis with weakness and tachycardia.

c. metabolic acidosis with muscle twitching and tremors.

d. metabolic alkalosis with nausea, vomiting, and convulsions.

c
Comprehension
Assessment
Physiological:
Physiological
Adaptation

48-15 The initial physical examination of an individual's fluid, electrolyte, and acid-base balance includes a focused assessment of the:

a. gastrointestinal system.

b. musculoskeletal system.

c. skin and mucous membranes.

d. heart and lungs.

c
Comprehension
Implementation
Physiological:
Physiological
Adaptation

48-16 When weighing a client with a nursing diagnosis of Fluid Volume Excess, the nurse should:

a   weigh the client at least two hours after a meal.

b. balance the scale daily.

c. document the type of scale used.

d. weigh the client without clothing.

48-17 At 3:00 P.M. a client has 150 cc remaining in his IV bag. At 4:30 P.M. the nurse hangs a new 1000 cc bottle of IV fluid and when she checks it at 10:15 P.M., there is 700 cc left. In addition, during the nurse's shift, the client drinks two 240 cc cartons of milk and 250 cc of water. He has had a liquid stool measuring 350 cc and has voided three times: 260 cc, 310 cc, and 175 cc. Which of the following should the nurse record on her I and O sheet?

a. intake = 940 cc; output = 745 cc

b. intake = 1,340 cc; output = 745 cc

c. intake = 1,180 cc; output = 1,095 cc

d. intake = 1,640 cc; output = 1,095 cc

48-18 Which of the following clinical signs is indicative of phlebitis at the IV site?

a. coolness

b. pallor

c. bleeding

d. warmth

48-19 The physician has ordered parenteral fluids, 1,000 ml of D LR in eight hours. The IV tubing box states the drip factor is 20 drops/ml. How many drops per minute should infuse?

a. 30

b. 40

c. 50

d. 60

48-20 During her initial assessment of a client, the nurse observes that his IV solution is not infusing. Which of the following should be her first intervention?

a. Inspect the tubing for kinks.

b. Notify the physician.

c. Discontinue the IV infusion.

d. Lower the height of the IV-solution container.

48-21 Ten minutes after the nurse begins a packed red blood cell transfusion, the client complains of chest pain and chills. His temperature is 102° F. Which of the following interventions should the nurse initiate first?

a. Slow the transfusion to a 'keep open' rate.

b. Notify the physician.

c. Stop the transfusion immediately.

d. Administer Tylenol as ordered for fever.

b
Knowledge
Implementation
Physiological:
Pharmacological and
Parenteral Therapies

48-22   Total parental nutrition (TPN) is administered through a central vein because TPN solution is:

    a.   isotonic.

    b.   hypertonic.

    c.   hypotonic.

    d.   atonic.

d
Application
Assessment
Physiological:
Physiological
Adaptation

48-23   A client has been admitted to the medical unit with a medical diagnosis of dehydration secondary to diuretic therapy. What nursing physical assessment criteria would the nurse expect to find?

    a.   distended neck and peripheral veins

    b.   increased blood pressure with clear breath sounds

    c.   fill bounding pulse with increased rate

    d.   dry mucous membranes with decreased salivation

b
Comprehension
Assessment
Physiological:
Physiological
Adaptation

48-24   A client's weight has increased in one day by approximately two pounds. The nurse knows that this increase in weight equal approximately how much fluid?

    a.   500 cc

    b.   1 L

    c.   300 ml

    d.   2 L

a
Application
Implementation
Physiological: Basic
Care and Comfort

48-25   The physician has placed a client on a fluid restriction of 1000 ml/24 hours. In helping the client maintain this fluid restriction, the nurse should:

    a.   provide client with fluids she prefers.

    b.   suggest sucking on hard candy.

    c.   provide the client with large containers of fluid.

    d.   remind the client frequently that her fluid is restricted.

c
Application
Implementation
Physiological:
Pharmacological and
Parenteral Therapies

48-26   After removing a intravenous catheter the nurse notices that tip has broken off, and it can be palpated at the site. What should the nurse do first?

    a.   Assess the client for respiratory complications.

    b.   Notify the physician immediately.

    c.   Apply a tourniquet above the insertion site.

    d.   Remove the tip with a scalpel.

b
Comprehension
Assessment
Physiological:
Physiological
Adaptation

48-27 A client has been admitted to the medical unit with a medical diagnosis of metabolic acidosis secondary to diabetes mellitus. Which of the following physical assessment criteria validates this diagnosis?

a. decreased respiratory rate and depth

b. fruity breath with deep, rapid respirations

c. tetany and hypertonic muscles

d. positive Trousseau's sign